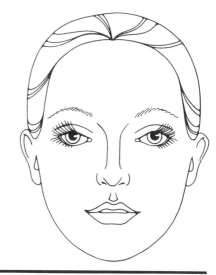

MAKEOVERS

Also by the author:

WRINKLES: *How to Prevent Them, How to Erase Them*
(with Lida Livingston)

Constance Schrader

MAKE

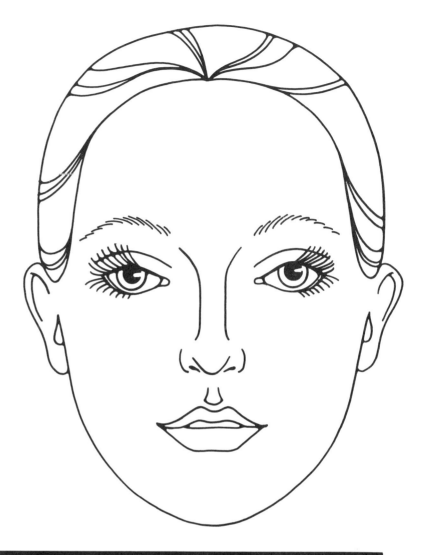

OVERS

With Illustrations by Glee LoScalzo

Prentice-Hall, Inc., Englewood Cliffs, New Jersey

Makeovers by Constance Schrader
Copyright © 1979 by Constance Schrader
All rights reserved. No part of this book may be
reproduced in any form or by any means, except
for the inclusion of brief quotations in a review,
without permission in writing from the publisher.
Printed in the United States of America
Prentice-Hall International, Inc., London
Prentice-Hall of Australia, Pty. Ltd., Sydney
Prentice-Hall of Canada, Ltd., Toronto
Prentice-Hall of India Private Ltd., New Delhi
Prentice-Hall of Japan, Inc., Tokyo
Prentice-Hall of Southeast Asia Pte. Ltd., Singapore
Whitehall Books Limited, Wellington, New Zealand
10 9 8 7 6 5 4 3 2

Library of Congress Cataloging in Publication Data
Schrader, Constance
Makeovers.

Bibliography: p.
1. Cosmetics.   I. Title.
RA778.S335 1979   646.7′2   79-4624
ISBN 0-13-545608-8

Dedicated to Lida Livingston

I want to thank my editor Dennis Fawcett,
production editor Edna Boschen, copyeditor Ilene McGrath,
art director Hal Siegel and designer Linda Huber.
Special thanks to my typist and friend-critic Jean Brown.

CONTENTS

PREFACE

This book is an entire course for practicing and perfecting your makeup techniques, using a composite portrait of your own face, drawn on a clear sheet of plastic. For the first time you will be able to see your face with the objectivity of an artist, and use that new vision to make yourself more beautiful.

The book is divided into two parts. Part One will show you how to study your features and identify and create the effects that enhance them. It will help you to bring out the good, and to camouflage or divert attention from the less than perfect. Using the plastic Beauty Palette, you can practice endlessly, experimenting with new looks, with your own or different cosmetics.

Part Two provides a complete selection of makeovers for changing or improving your appearance. Regardless of what age or type you are, whether you're a career woman or housewife or still in school, a makeover can help you achieve the right look for you. There are specially developed "celebrity charts" in this section that will help you identify your special type and show you how to achieve the makeover you want for any occasion.

Don't hesitate to explore new face designs and effects. A beautiful world of admiration and success is waiting. If you really want it, it can be yours.

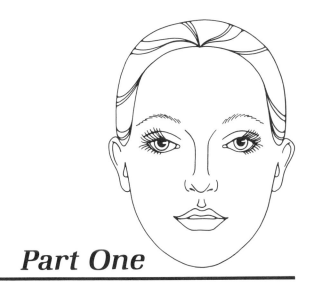

Part One

MAKEUP

USING THE BEAUTY PALETTE

Unlike most beauty books, this one is a workbook; you are supposed to color in it. It is designed to use with your own makeup.

Bound into the book (page 32) is a plastic sheet or Beauty Palette, on which you will draw your composite portrait. If you flip through the following pages, you'll notice that there are line drawings showing facial features of various sizes and shapes. To make the composite portrait of yourself, you position features similar to yours on a face shape that is also similar to yours. From the line drawings you select the features that most nearly match your own. On the Beauty Palette, trace the features, creating your composite portrait. Now, practicing with your own makeup, you can learn to perfect your features on a face that actually looks like you.

To get an idea of how to draw your look-alike face, start with the beautifully shaped mouth below.

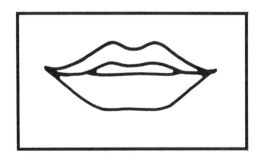

Place the plastic over these lips. Using your own lipstick—tube, pot of gloss, sponge gloss, or pencil— trace the outline of the lips on the plastic. If you make a mistake, don't worry. With a tissue and some cold cream, or a dab of soap and water, you can clean the plastic easily.

Just as you've traced the shape of these lips, you can trace the shape of every one of your own features and apply makeup on them.

1 Select all of your facial features from the drawings supplied. Trace them in the appropriate place on the Beauty Palette, using a very soft pencil, a grease pencil, or best of all, a light tan eyebrow pencil.
2 Paint and color in each feature with your own cosmetics.
3 Use a piece of light tan paper, pink paper, or even cream white paper under the Beauty Palette to match your own skin color and to make the individual features look neater.

The features provided for selection include eyebrows, eyes, noses, lips, and also basic face shapes. All the features are normal size for a woman about 5 feet, 6 inches tall, with a head about 7½ inches long. Naturally, face sizes vary and you'll have to adjust the face shape to reflect your own size. However, the features provided are suitable for most people.

Let's practice on one of your own features. Turn to page 47 and look at the five lip shapes shown: full lips; lips that are out of proportion or misshaped; unevenly colored lips; lips that are too full, and lips that are too thin. Select the lips that most resemble yours. Then, on a thin piece of paper, a piece of waxed paper, or other transparent paper, trace the lip shape.

Place the traced lip shape under the Beauty Palette. Using lipstick or lip pencil, fill in the lips. You are now ready to learn how to improve their shape and contour.

In the same way you can trace all your features and learn how to perfect thcm.

YOUR FACE SHAPE

The proportions of your face as well as the position of the features can make your face seem balanced and beautiful. The proportions below are what are usually accepted as a good guide.

The distance between the top of the head and the top of the nose should be about the same as the distance between the nose and the bottom tip of the chin. The width of the jaw and forehead and their shape also have an effect on the total face shape. The oval face, with the forehead slightly wider than the jawline, is considered ideal.

The actual shape of your face is dependent on your bone structure; the shape of your jawbone and forehead really determine how you will look. But you can use makeup to create light and shadow areas that will make your face look like a perfect oval.

Just as stage makeup is based on the use of light and shadow to create special effects, your everyday makeup can use the same scientific optical methods for ac-

tually reshaping your face or parts of it. You can apply light colors to reflect light and make your features or parts of a feature advance and seem larger, or use dark to make features retreat and seem smaller.

Painters use shadow colors of umber and grey, but if you used those colors on your face they would just make your face look dirty. Skin colors are the most subtle and seem to work best for sculpturing with your makeup. One foundation in a color slightly darker than your own skin color, and another in a color lighter than your own skin, work much better than thick opaque coversticks. The coversticks seem to goo and always cake after a few hours.

Besides a darker and lighter foundation, you should have a series of shadows that are available as eye shadows and as rouge. These come in either powder or creme form. The powder is best for normal and oily skins, the creme shadow or blusher is best for dry skin. There is makeup that is specially made for black skin, and stage makeup also will provide a large variety of shades, tints, and hues. The most important factor is the craftswomanship with which the colors are applied.

Experiment with light and dark, but always remember the basic rule: makeup darker than skin diminishes the flaw; makeup lighter than skin calls attention to the lightened section. It is a rule that is used over and over again.

14

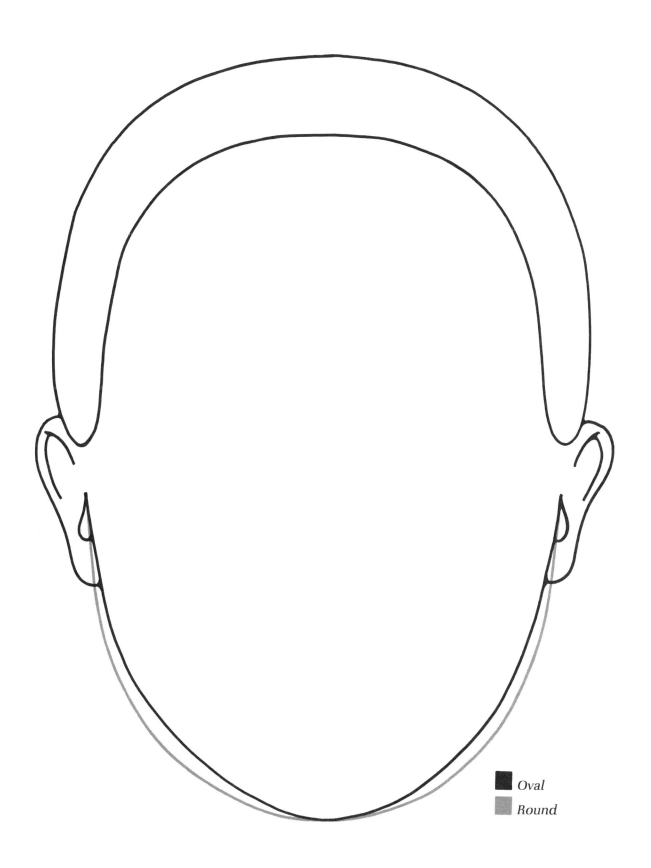

Oval
Round

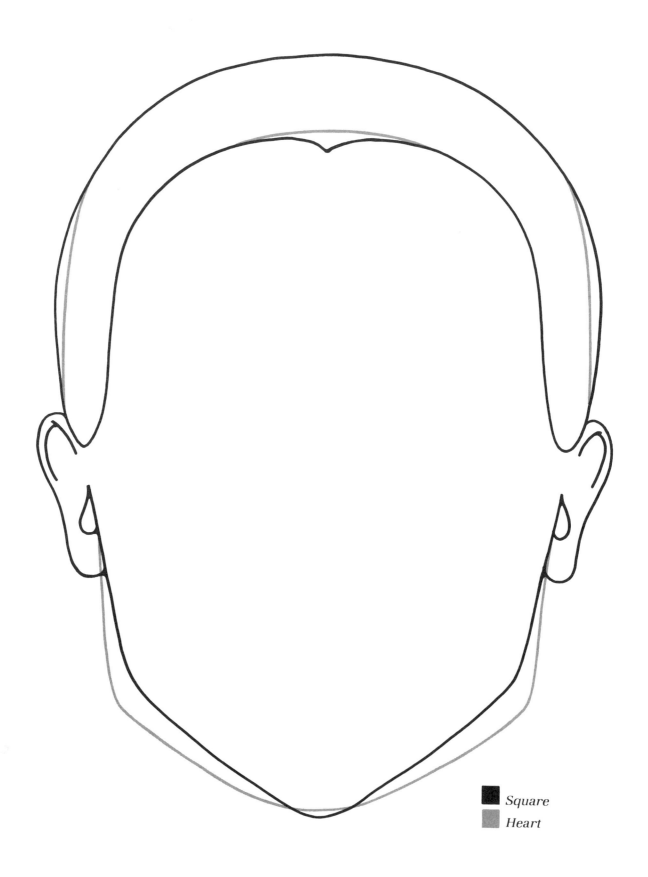

Square

Heart

Pin your hair back and wash and dry your face carefully. Read the descriptions of face shapes that follow and then, from the illustrated face shapes, select the one that is most like your own. You'll notice that there are three different shapes on two pages. No one is exactly one shape or another; try to select the face that is closest to your exact shape.

Now trace the face shape on the plastic Beauty Palette. Once the face is traced, you might want to draw lines on either side of the face to look like a neck. They should start even with the outer corner of eye, and be drawn from the jaw.

Oval Face   You are lucky. Play up your best feature with a simple hair style. If you have a small, well-shaped nose, keep your hair away from your temples and jaw; dramatize your eyes.

Round Jaw, Round Cheeks   Your jaws are round in shape and your face is rather wide. Your cheeks and forehead are rounded and full too. This face shape can have a rounded or pointed chin, but usually the chin is small.

Your eyebrows should be wing-shaped, pointing upward and outward toward the temples.

A shading, darker than normal, in a line from the outer corner of each eye, down the cheek to be level with the tip of the nose and up over the temple to the hairline should be blended well with the normal foundation color.

Square Jaw, Square Forehead
In profile, the jaw and the chin are on the same line, and there is almost a right angle formed by the jawbone. The chin is usually small, with the mouth often wide and low-seeming on the chin.

Keep eyebrows round and play up eyes rather than mouth. Lengthen chin with a light shade from lip downward.

Sculpt the jaw by shading the angle section on the lower cheeks, below the ear. If the forehead is square, darken the corners of the temples, near the hairline, and blend well.

Avoid square necks or hats placed squarely on your head; they repeat the angle of the jaw.

Heart-Shaped, with Wide Forehead and Pointed Jaw   Many people find this shape most attractive. Play up your eyes. But if they are too widely set, use heavy liner on upper and lower lids from the inner corner to the middle of the eye.

You can make the jaw look wider by covering the outer cheek with a light shade and rounding out the pointed chin with a dab of dark shadow. The temples can be narrowed with dark shadow on the sides of the forehead.

Avoid V-neck blouses, or pendants; they repeat the line of your pointed chin.

Brunettes with heavy hair on the sides of the jaw might bleach the hair. You'll find that the light hair makes the jaw seem wider.

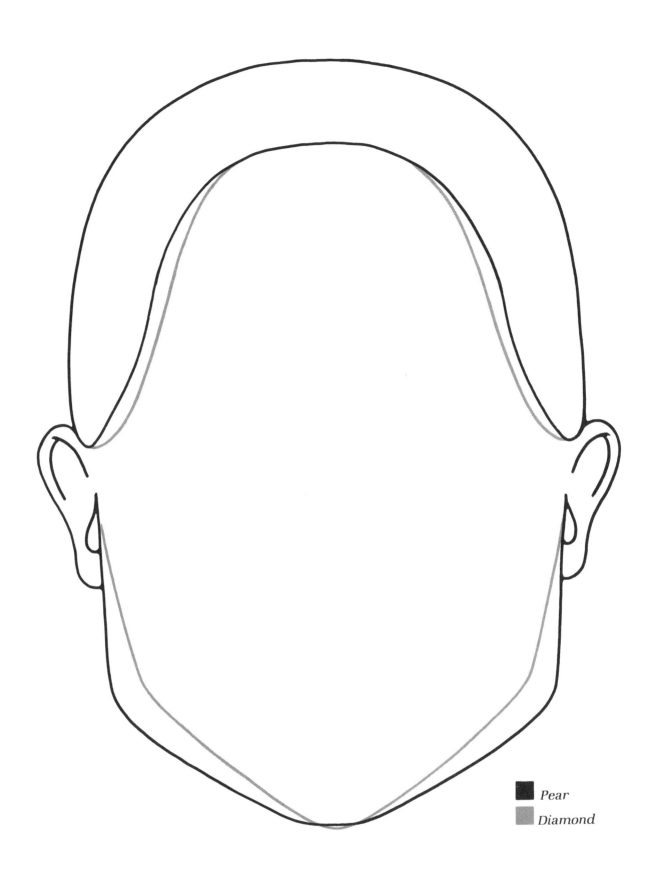

Pear

Diamond

Pear-Shaped with Narrow Forehead and Square or Heavy Jaw
Make your jaw seem more delicate by darkening the lower cheeks and dramatizing the cheekbones, by coloring below the cheekbone and highlighting above, near the outer eye.

Broaden the narrow forehead with light or reflective foundation blended to the hairline from the outer temple. And peak your brows as far as possible to the outer edges of the brow.

Low Forehead, Long Jaw Raise your forehead by lightening the top of your forehead near the hairline, or obscuring the hairline with bangs.

Shorten the jaw and chin by shading the bottom of the jaw and chin. Draw attention to the eyes and central section of the face.

Soften the jawline with wide cowl necklines and draped scarves.

Long Face with Narrow Forehead and Cheeks, and Pointed or Long Chin To shorten the look of a long face, you will have to bring the sides of the face forward visually. This is done by using a lighter than skin shade. It is also important to shorten the forehead and the chin with a shadow slightly darker than skin shade. The chin and hairline need a dark foundation, or dark blusher blended carefully.

If you are a brunette, you should bleach the hair on the sides of your cheeks near the jaw and also at the hairline. The bleach will lighten the soft downy hair and will actually make your face look broader. If the downy hair is no problem, or after you have it bleached, wear your hair back and show your ears. Keep some interest just about the level of the top of your ear. This can be done with ornamental combs or barrettes.

Diamond Face, with Narrow Forehead and Pointed Chin, Wide at Temples Just as with the long face, shorten the chin and forehead slightly with shadow darker than skin color. You might want to experiment with changing your hairline. You can depilatorize the sides of the forehead and see if you like the effect. George Masters, the famous Hollywood makeup artist, changed the shape of Luci Johnson Nugent's face by actually shaving her hairline—on the very evening of Luci's White House wedding. Broaden the jawline with light-reflecting blusher drawn in a line around the curve of the jaw, but not on the chin.

Weak Chin Apply a lighter than normal shade on the center tip of your chin, and extend it to the jaws on each side of your face.

Double Chin The underside of the chin and upper neck should be darkened slightly with foundation.

Ears Too Large Darken them slightly with foundation and a dusting of blusher.

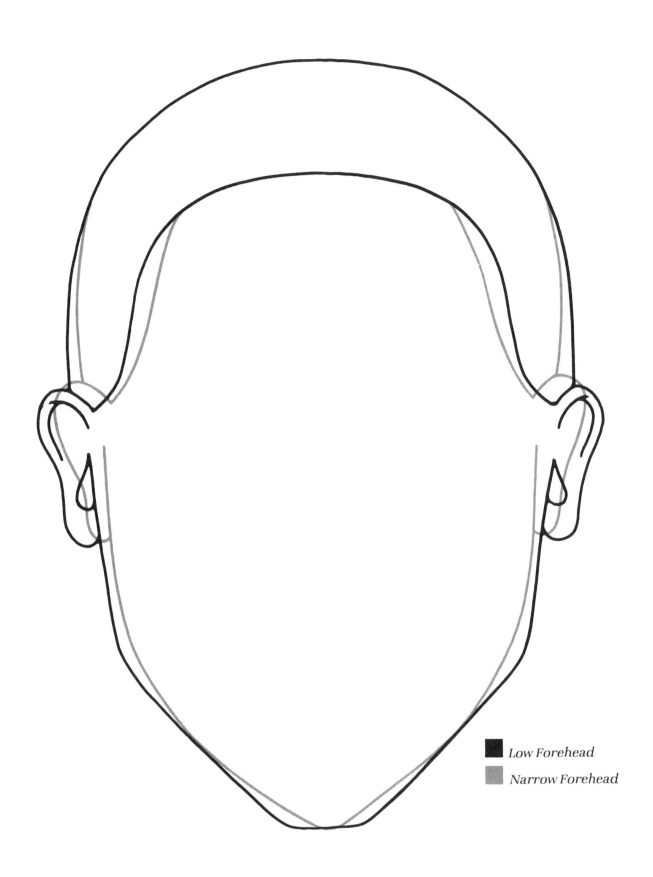

■ Low Forehead

■ Narrow Forehead

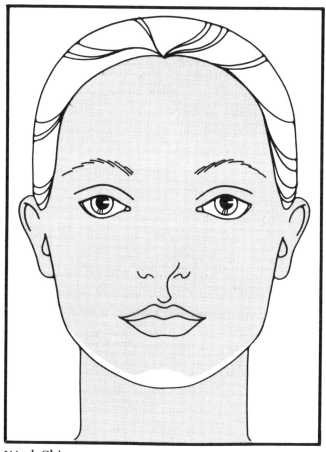

Weak Chin

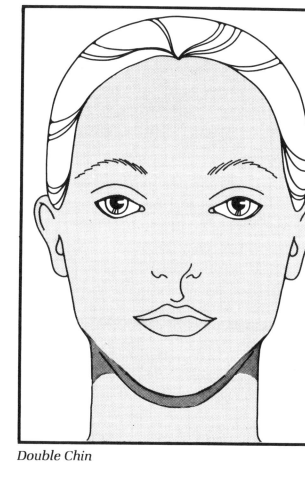

Double Chin

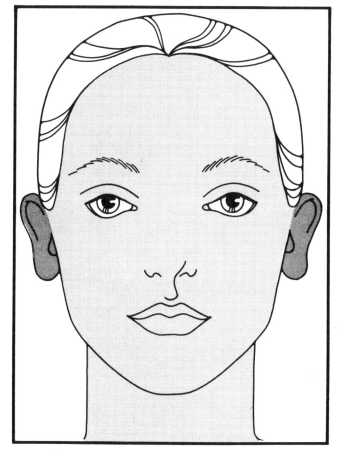

Large Ears

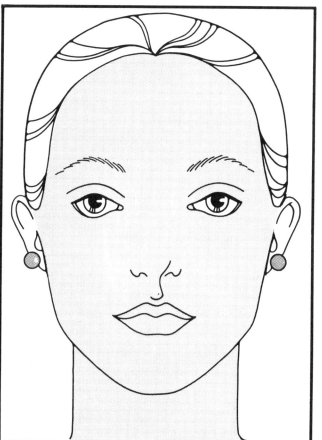

Small Ears

Ears Too Small, No Lobes

Lighten the ears and make them seem more prominent with large earrings that cover the tiny lobes. If the upper part of the ear is too small or badly formed, a line of light can make the contours seem more even.

Uneven Face, One Side Wider Than the Other

No one has a perfectly symmetrical face. To see which side of your face is wider, do the following:

1 Draw your hair back and stand in front of the mirror.
2 Take a piece of plain white paper.
3 Cover one side of the face at a time. It will be easy to see the difference between the two sides.
4 Place the paper so that you can see only your eyes and forehead. Note which eye is higher if they are uneven.

Most people will find that one side of the face seems older than the other. The side that ages most quickly is probably the side on which you rest your weight when sleeping. Special care should be taken to sleep on your back so that the blood supply reaches both sides of your face evenly.

Adapt your makeup. Apply blusher to each side of your face—lighten the narrow side; darken the wider side.

CHEEKS

A pinkish glow at the cheeks indicates good health, and rouge is probably· the oldest of the cosmetics. Fashions in cheek colors can change from season to season and year to year, but you should always use a shade that is flattering to your skin tone—no matter what fashion dictates. Purple and orange shades are not usually good for blondes, and orange-brown shades make many olive-skinned brunettes look grimy. Colors suitable for pink-toned skins should be in the rose-peach family. Darker skins look best in the rose-grape tones.

Rouge should be applied after the face contouring is complete, but it can also be used to enhance the shadowing of features.

In Europe, rouge is usually applied to the cheekbone or the fullest part of the cheek. In America, it is most often applied on the lower part of the cheekbone or beneath the bone, where the face sinks slightly to the top roots of the upper molars.

The cheekbones are roundish in shape, something like the size and shape of a walnut shell. Think of half of a walnut shell under your skin below the corner of your eye. The top of the shell catches the light; the bottom of the shell near the seam is darker because it is in the shadow. This is normal since sunlight and most electric lighting is from above, not below.

It is important that rouge be blended very carefully—imperceptibly into the makeup base. Otherwise you can end up with a clownish look. Many people use rouge for a sculpture or contour makeup. There is nothing wrong with

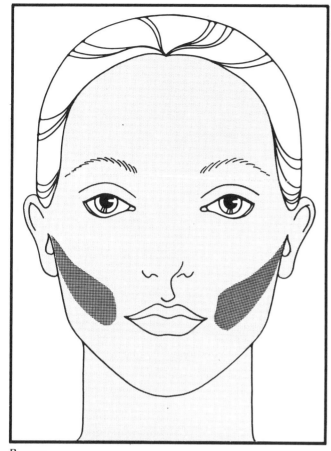

Rouge

that, if you are an expert and can get a natural effect, but remember that they are quite different. Rouge is an imitation of natural high color, whereas facial contour colors are imitations of shadows. Worse than *no* makeup is the current vogue for many young women who wear a model's camera makeup on the streets: an orange-brown shape of color from mid-ear to mouth, a diagonal blotch!

If you have sunken cheeks, wear a light makeup mid-cheek below the cheekbone and a light pinkish rouge directly on the high point of the cheekbone. It will give your face a healthy glow and lift.

If your face is round or square, keep rouge away from the ears. If your face is narrow, keep rouge away from the nose.

SKIN PERFECTION

Foundation

The purpose of a foundation is to protect and enhance the skin. The skin of the face and neck can and should be covered with a foundation almost all the time. Some skins even benefit from tinted medicinal foundation worn when sleeping. The right water-based foundation will dry out oily skin, cover blemishes, and promote healing; for other types of skin, an oil-based foundation will protect the skin from cold, sun, and wind. You should have a complete wardrobe of foundations in different

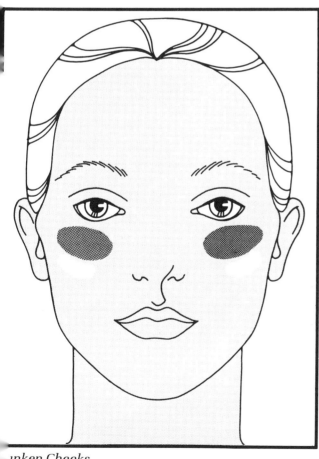

Sunken Cheeks

23

textures and different shades. You can and should use a variety of foundations to even out the changes in your natural skin tones and textures. My foundation supply includes white, ivory, beige, yellow, and tan colors in water-soluble liquid, oil-based liquid, and cake form. It is best to begin with only a few shades and textures and see what is most attractive and convenient for you. Foundations come in a great variety of cremes, liquids, and cakes.

Liquid base is the easiest to use and the most popular. The water-soluble foundation is best for oily skins. It usually comes in a larger bottle than the oil-based foundation and must be thoroughly shaken before using.

Apply with fingers. The oil-based liquid is very easy to use; simply dot on and even out with the fingertips.

Medicated base liquids have become popular for blemished and oily skins, but be sure that the medication does not cause an allergic reaction. As with any medication, the side effects can often be more unpleasant than the problem.

Hypo-allergenic makeups are compounded without the ingredients that most commonly cause an allergic reaction. This term has been dropped from most cosmetics because it is difficult—probably impossible—to exclude every substance that is irritating to everyone.

Souffle, whipped or fluffy creme is very popular for people who have smooth, unlined skin with few blemishes or discolorations. It gives very little coverage but it is easy to apply because of the light consistency, and it is only slightly oily.

Gels or stains provide translucent coverage, a color coat with almost no opacity. It hides nothing. Gels are popular for outdoor and vacation wear; it will give you an instant tan or flush. Because it dries so quickly, it can be difficult to apply unless you cover your face with water and moisturizer. This is one makeup foundation you cannot dot on and then spread. In just an instant you will have dry spots of color. When applying, dot and blend the dot immediately. Your fingers will become quite stained, but the gel washes off easily.

Matte base comes in a tube and combines a creme base with the powder. It offers good coverage but it has a tendency to clog pores and to cake; also, when applied to a lined face, it cracks and draws attention to wrinkles and dry skin.

Pressed powder can be used for a foundation in an emergency. It is convenient for travel and quick touch-ups. But touch-ups are make-do measures. Pressed powder has many of the drawbacks of the matte-base foundation.

Creme stick foundation comes in what looks like a huge lipstick tube. It is oily, and a waxy base is the main ingredient, so it is not recommended for oily skin. There is a slightly less solid version that comes in small pots or wide-necked jars; this is easier to spread than the sticks. It is very opaque; a creme foundation in a lighter than skin color makes an excellent contour cream for dry skins.

Cake base comes in large, flat, pancake-looking containers and is applied with a large damp sponge. Max Factor, the famous Hollywood makeup artist, developed it in the 1930's for movie stars, and the Max Factor brand still makes the most popular and, to me, the best of this kind. It covers even oily skin and it doesn't melt away. It is not recommended for dry or lined skin, though. A wet cotton ball can be used instead of a sponge for application. The sponge must be carefully washed after each use.

Apply your foundation as quickly as possible with upward and outward motions. Try not to pull or drag the skin. If your skin is less than firm and/or lined, hold the section of skin you are working on taut, by tightening the muscles, opening your mouth, or puffing out your cheeks.

Be sure that a thick, smooth cover of moisturizer is applied before your foundation.

Moisturizers

A moisturizer is one of the many emollients that are used to coat the dry surface cells of the skin; while it is softening the skin it is also preventing the skin's natural moisturizer—water—from escaping. The best and most effective moisturizer is water. Night creams, hand creams, skin creams, and body unguents in liquid, lotion, and drop form all are designed to preserve the skin's moisture.

After washing your face, when your skin is still wet, apply a moisturizer before using any other cosmetic. Also, during the day, freshen your makeup by spraying and misting with water.

Tinted moisturizers contain small amounts of suspended pigments that are designed to react with the color of your skin. Use the following guideline:

1 Sallow skin: Brighten it with blue or lavender.
2 Ruddy skin: Tone it down with green or bluish-green.
3 Dark, sallow skin: It reacts well with apricot.
4 Black skin: It seems to hold foundation color better if a blue tint moisturizer is used.

A tinted moisturizer, along with contour cremes, blushers, and shadows, should enable you to create the smooth and flawless background for your perfect features.

POWDER

When your foundation is perfectly applied—your shadow and blusher have been applied so that every feature is shaped to perfection and your face has a balanced proportion—it is time to think about powder. If you use a creme blusher or rouge, you will apply it *before* powdering; if you use a powder blusher (and if your face is oily, this is the one for you), then blusher comes *after* powder.

Powder is like a beauty veil: it sets the foundation, blends all colors, and protects other makeup; the soft velvet is the perfect finishing touch. Powder is in many forms—loose, pressed into a cake, combined with foundation—and it comes in white, color, and transparent gossamer shadings.

Loose powder is the most popular. It is finely pulverized and can remove the "shine" from the face. Talc is the main ingredient in most face powder, but clay, zinc oxides, and colorings are also included. Potato starch and cornstarch are sometimes also used.

Translucent loose powder reflects light more than other powders. It contains a larger amount of titanium dioxide than other powders, and is actually quite opaque.

A light dusting of powder is transparent, but the thicker the coating of powder the less transparent. Powders that are transparent are very fine and cover the skin very lightly.

Pressed powders are sometimes used for quick touch-ups. The powder is combined with a small amount of foundation. This is not suitable for oily skin because it has a tendency to clog pores, and it isn't suitable for dry skin because it has a tendency to cake.

Matte foundations which usually come in tubes, are advertised as combining foundation and powder. It is similar to pressed powder and is very opaque. Some people find it useful for covering blemishes.

Apply powder in one or more light coats, delicately dusting it on. Use as many coats as you wish, but be sure it doesn't go on so thick in some places that it cakes. Many people like to use cotton balls or a wad of soft absorbent cotton as an applicator. The most effective powder brush I've ever used is a beaver-fur shaving brush. However, it required constant washing and was often too damp to use. Some people use pastry brushes or feathers—both work well and are inexpensive.

EYES

The next chart shows four basic eye shapes. If you study these eye shapes, you will find one that most resembles your own eye shape. Look in the mirror. Are both of your eyes the same size? The same shape? Is one eye slightly larger, slightly more open, perhaps on a different level?

Place the eye illustration under the plastic Beauty Palette and align the eyes separately so each in turn is positioned as your eyes are on your face. The eyes that are closest to the shape of your own eyes should be positioned under the plastic in the appropriate spot on the face. The eyes will be traced one eye at a time.

The eyes in the illustration are a bit large. This is so you can adjust each eye shape to your own shape within the basic outline. Do trace slightly inside the outline.

Use your dark eyeliner pencil—black for brunettes and black women; brown or auburn for blondes and redheads. Trace the eye shape carefully on the plastic surface. If you make a mistake, simply wipe it clean with a bit of cold cream and a tissue. Or, you can sponge mistakes away with soap and water.

Now you can step back and look at your tracing. Your eyes should be outlined on the plastic against the background of the correct skin tone. Don't worry about the lashes; concentrate on the outline.

You are now ready to start practicing your own special beauty techniques, right on the plastic. You will want to paint or color with your own shadow and your own pencils. If your powder is dry, it might not immediately stick to the plastic. You can make it adhere by placing an undercoat of foundation on the eyelid and eye area.

On the following pages are beauty tips on how to change and enhance each of the eye shapes. Remember that each eye can be made up separately to make it look perfect. In this way you can create the illusion that your eyes are symmetrical, even if they are not.

Eye Tools

It is said that eyes are the mirror of your soul: they can be laughing, flashing, alluring, loving, tender, or understanding. They are blue, green, brown, grey, black, gold-specked, orange, or violet. The shape, the size, and the distance between your eyes are very important!

In order to perfect and enhance your eyes' shape and color, you'll need some basic beauty tools.

1 Pencils or liquid liner with its own brush
2 A sharpener
3 An eyebrow brush
4 Eye shadow in liquid or powder form, or crayons of color
5 Mascara in cake or liquid form
6 Tweezers
7 Toothpicks to separate mascara-stuck lashes
8 Q-Tips
9 Cotton to wrap on toothpicks to make your own Q-Tips or clean away makeup
10 Eye oil (light, thin vegetable oil)
11 A soothing eyewash

Remember to be very gentle with the skin around your eyes, and, of course, never put anything in your eyes. Pat colors on rather than smoothing them or rubbing them. Always apply moisturizer to the eye area before makeup. And blot: do not wipe away makeup when you want to remove it.

Small Eyes Small eyes should never be outlined; outlining just defines them and makes them look smaller. A delicate series of dots that can be applied with a very sharp soft pencil, or dotted on with a liner brush, is best. Keep the line at the base of the top lashes

Small Eyes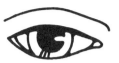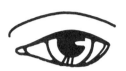

Round Eyes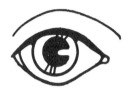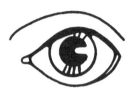

Hanging Lids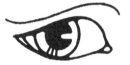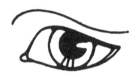

Deep Set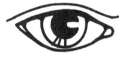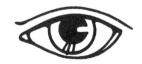

only. An outline of white or light blue should be applied to the inner ledge of the lid; it will seem to extend the eye white.

The lids should be kept very light, and the darker shadow color should extend from the crease upward and outward to the top of the eyebrow.

Use a heavy coating of mascara on the tips of both the upper and lower lashes. Powder the tip and wait; then apply mascara for a second coat.

Round Eyes Round eyes can be slightly extended to make them appear wider and less bulging. Extend the eye slightly with a pencil line drawn in a triangle on the outer edge of the eye. It should be no more than ¼ of an inch. Fill in the tiny skin triangle with very light beige or white.

Spread your shadow across the outer edge of the eye, and continue it past the small drawn triangle and around its lower edge. None of this should be harsh; the color should be smudged slightly.

Avoid extreme arches in your eyebrow. Do not pluck the brow to a round crescent shape. Keep the brow fairly dark and rather straight.

Overhanging Eyelids When the skin below the eyebrow pouches slightly, you will want to lift it and open the entire eye area. This is most common in the eye that is over 40 years old, and it can be aging.

Place the shadow on the in-side corner of the eye and over the entire inner section of the lid. It should be very soft and not too dark, since that would have the effect of bringing the eyes together and create a shadow around the bridge of the nose. Then place a lighter color shadow below the brow to the outer part of the eye. This will open the outer corner of the eye and make the soft sagging skin seem less evident.

Keep the brows light and well tended. Trim brows with scissors so that hairs do not overhang and add to that drooping effect.

Deep-set Eyes Use lighter than skin color shadow around the eye, on the eyelids, and in the crease that marks the meeting of the eyelid and the skin of the brow bone. Directly under the brow, on the brow bone, use a rather dark shadow. Browns and greys seem to work well under the brow after a pearly cream-white has been smoothed over the lid.

Use mascara only on the tip ends of the lashes and do not use eyeliner.

Narrow, Squinty Eyes Open the eye in the middle by lining the inner lid with white, light blue, or violet. Extend the eye slightly at the outer corner with a dark liner from the outer end to slightly beyond the eye, both top and bottom.

Apply a dot of light to the center lid and extend it upward toward the brow.

Apply a medium blue, grey, or

beige only on the outer edge of the eyebrow.

You've just seen how the five most common eye beauty flaws can be corrected. The next eye types are less common, but just as easily overcome or featured.

Eyes Too Close Together Use light or white sculpture on the sides of the nose and around the inner corner of the eye. Darken only the very outer corners. Bring eyebrow slightly beyond the outer corner of the eye.

Bland or Pale Color Apply a color contrasting the color of your eye color. If it is a very light blue, spice or nut brown is a good contrast; a cloudy brown eye will look clearer when surrounded by marine blue or violet.

Feature Almond or Slanted Eyes Heavily line the lower lid and bring the line slightly up and past the outer edge of the eye. Apply a deep color to upper lid's outer edge. Use several heavy coats of mascara on the top and bottom lashes.

Bags Under Eyes Balance the light-reflecting puffy bags by lightening the upper lids and brow bone area. Brush brows up and draw attention to the hairline. Apply light to the creases under the eyes.

Are your eyes your best feature? Would you like to play up their color, shape, and depth? Here is how to enhance your beautiful eyes:

The upper lids should be wrapped in color and the color brought around the outer edge of the eye to the bottom lids. A light or pale highlight on the brow bone is shaded into the colored lid. Then, the lash bases are all dotted with a tiny row of smudged and softened lines.

A thick coating of mascara should cover both the upper and lower lashes.

Eyeliner

Eyeliners are used to accentuate or change the actual shape of your eyes. They are usually available as pencils, liquid, cake form (applied with a very thin, tiny sable brush), or a newer pencil brush. Eyeliner can be used with shadow, with mascara, with both, or alone. Waterproof liner must be removed with oil or a cream.

The most popular colors are brown, charcoal, and black, but brownish-wine, plum, and blue-grey are becoming very popular.

The eyeliner should be applied at the roots of the lashes, or as near as possible to the very base of the lashes. Don't extend the line beyond the inner corner of the eye, and never extend it in thick wings over the outer eyelids; it is old-fashioned looking and actually makes your eyes look smaller. Correctly applied, eyeliner can

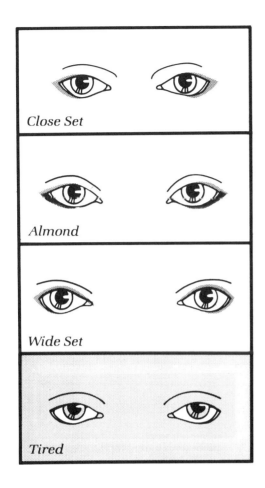

Close Set

Almond

Wide Set

Tired

1 close-set, stop slightly before the center of the eye.
2 almond-shaped, make the bottom line darker than the top.
3 wide-set, line the full top lid and the outer half of the lid on the bottom.
4 bloodshot or tired, try a white or blue line on the inner ledge of the lower lid.

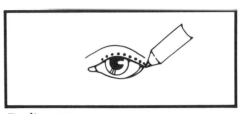

Eyeliner Dot

One of the newest techniques in applying eyeliner is to dot the liner rather than draw it in a smooth unbroken line. You might also smudge each dot slightly. To smudge the liner, use a flat toothpick with one end wrapped in a tiny bit of cotton. (Obviously a new one is needed for each application to avoid bacteria growth.) This technique works well for pencil eyeliner, but does not work for liquid liner.

Using an eyeliner pencil is an easy and natural way to draw on the plastic Beauty Palette. You would be using the pencils just as you use them on your skin. A black, dark brown, or medium brown pencil is best.

It will take a bit of concentration to draw on your lashes, because they are one of the few features that you cannot duplicate on the plastic exactly as they are on your face. But having the plastic

really make ordinary eyes look fabulous.

Liner is a bit tricky, and there are ways of making a neat, mistake-proof line more easily. Place a small mirror or a hand mirror flat on a table or a level surface that is even with the bottom of your nose. Look downward, through your lashes; you should be able to see your upper lid and the base of your lashes in the mirror.

Start at the outer corner and work inward. Do not, as most directions tell you, hold or pull your lid taut. Just draw a line inward toward the inner end of the top lid. If your eyes are:

as a guide will help you visualize some of the effects possible.

Mascara

Many women consider mascara their most important cosmetic. It really can do more for the morale, and for an ultra-luxurious look, than any other cosmetic. Mascara comes in many forms:

Cake comes in small rectangles with small brushes for application. Many people think this is best; you can moisten the cake and get exactly the consistency you want. But you should *never* wet the cake with saliva, and you should wash the brush carefully after each use.

Creme mascara is sold in small tubes. It is nice and thick, and many women find it gives good coverage although it has a tendency to gob on lash tips.

Liquid is sold in small bottles with tiny comb applicators; several coats are often needed.

Roll-on, in a thick liquid, with a spiral or straight brush applicator that fits in the dispenser, is the most popular.

Lash-builder mascaras contain tiny filaments almost like the plush of velvet, which are cut free and suspended in the colored liquid. These tiny fibers stick to the lashes when the mascara dries and make the lashes thick and furry.

Waterproof mascara must be removed with oil.

Eyelash dyes and eyebrow dyes are made of highly purified chemical dyes. They are in limited colors. They must be used only by pro-

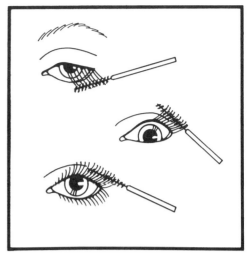

Mascara

fessionals, and many people hesitate to use them because they fear allergic reactions.

Apply mascara to all of your lashes, upper and lower. Many people find the automatic spiral brush the easiest to use:

1 Lower your top lids about halfway. Apply mascara to the top side of the upper lid's lashes.
2 Then slightly tilt head back and open eyes wide. Apply mascara to the underside of the upper lashes.
3 Use an even stroke and bring the brush from the base to the tips.
4 Then, with the brush newly loaded, double and triple coat the tips of the lashes, spreading the mascara with a horizontal move from the tips of the lashes around the inner eye to the tips of the lashes at the outer eye. Repeat from the outer tips to the inner, several times.
5 Allow tip lashes to dry slightly.
6 Powder lashes very lightly and repeat mascara application.
7 Allow top lashes to dry completely.
8 Tilt the head forward slightly; look downward.
9 Coat only outer sides of the bottom lashes in the same way as the top,

first from base to tip, then tips only in a horizontal movement.

10 Finally coat both the upper and lower lashes, as a last touch.

If your lashes stick together or the mascara beads on the lashes, use a flat wooden toothpick to separate the lashes. Gently, using a slight sawing motion cut through the caked lashes. And do it immediately, before the mascara dries. If the mascara does dry, sticking the lashes together, wrap the end of the toothpick in cotton, wet the cotton (oil for waterproof mascara), and very gently melt the dry mascara and separate the lashes.

If your lower lashes curl onto your lower lids and dot them with the wet mascara, simply use a paper slip under your lashes as you apply the mascara. I like plain white paper cut in small pieces, or index cards.

It is a good idea to clean any mascara spots or mistakes immediately. The longer you wait, the more difficult cleanup becomes; and when mascara dries, it becomes almost impossible. However, I've found that a cotton-wrapped toothpick, used with a twirling motion, helps.

Eyelash Curlers

Many beauty experts, and almost all professional makeup artists who work with models, use eyelash curlers. They are not included here because of the hundreds of people I've talked to have had the same experience I've had: curlier, but fewer, eyelashes.

Fake Eyelashes

About fifteen years ago false eyelashes were considered part of every woman's makeup. Joan Crawford's estate included hundreds of pairs. Women have experimented with glues, fur, human hair, and a variety of techniques. The reason they are not included here is that false lashes must be applied with an adhesive. No matter how careful you are in removing the fake lashes, some of your own lashes lift off as well. In about six months many wearers *have* to depend on the artificial lashes—their own lids are bald!

EYEBROWS

Just as you selected the face shape that seemed most like your own, and the eye shape that seemed most like your own, now you will find the eyebrow shape that will best balance your face and focus on your eyes. Select the brows from the four basic shapes and place the brow shapes under the plastic Beauty Palette. With your eyeliner pencil, carefully trace the outline shape.

Now look in the mirror and then back to the plastic. Slightly feather the brows with hairlike pencil strokes so that the brows actually look "hairy."

Look at the picture. The eyes are exactly the same shape and the same distance apart; but notice how the brow shape affects the appearance of the eyes beneath

33

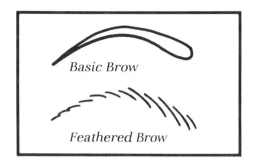

Basic Brow

Feathered Brow

the brows. Shaping the brows will highlight the eyes.

Shaggy, unruly, thin, uneven, or thick eyebrows are important to your total look. Disproportionate eyebrows can throw off the balance of an otherwise perfect face. Eyebrows can frame your eyes in a flattering manner and enhance your personality.

Shape and density of eyebrows change with style, and tweezed-to-a-line eyebrows may never grow back. Therefore, be careful and think before you tweeze.

When you do tweeze, you need the following tools:

1 cold cream or oil
2 cotton
3 tweezers
4 witch hazel or an astringent
5 brow brush
6 Vaseline or gloss
7 nail scissors
8 pencils or brush-on colors

A word of caution: don't pluck eyebrows from above—always from beneath the brow, to preserve the natural contour. Pluck each hair singly, in the direction in which it grows. Never pluck a clump at one time. Don't shave your brows; they will grow back in an unruly jungle.

You can trim long brow hairs with a nail scissors. Using a brow brush, feather the brows upward and trim evenly.

Using an eyebrow pencil, or a small eyebrow brush loaded with mascara, or pencil color, you can fill in bare spaces in your brows.

Your brow shape should follow the natural shape of the upper eye bone or brow bone. It should follow the line of your eyelid for a smooth consistent look of a perfect jewel in its setting. Always work with nature, if possible!

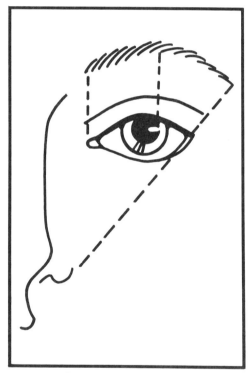

Brow Scale

Your eyebrow should start directly above the inner corner of the eye, right above the small triangle of flesh that is between the eyeball and the point where the upper and lower lids meet.

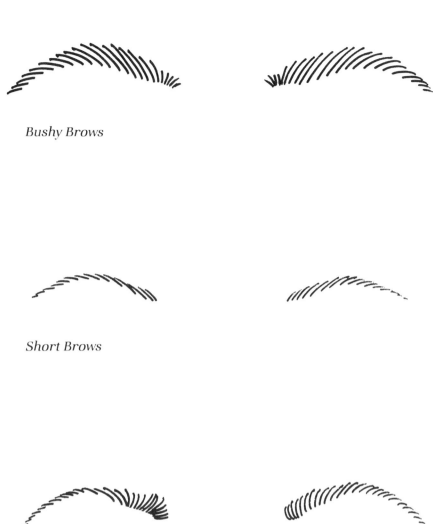

Bushy Brows

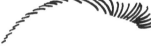

Short Brows

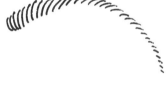

Uneven Brows

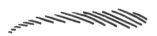

Straight Brows

The highest point of the eyebrow should be directly above the outer edge of the pupil, the center of the iris—the circle of color around the pupil—when you are looking directly ahead.

To locate where the brow should end, imagine a line drawn diagonally from the tip of the nostril (left nostril for left eye, right nostril for right eye) past the outer tip of the eye and extended upward toward the temple. The point where this imaginary line hits the eyebrows, should be the outer end of the brow.

Bushy Brows These brows grow below the bone, making the eye seem dark and heavy. Careful thinning and brushing can bring them up and open the entire eye area.

Short Brows This brow is well shaped and graceful, but too short for the eye. The brow should extend slightly beyond the outer corner of the eye. Extend the brow by continuing the line of the curve.

Uneven Brows Ragged, uneven brows give an unfinished look to any face. They overpower the eye and are not graceful. Arch the brow, extend and fill in any empty areas.

Straight Brows These brows often give a face a hurt or questioning expression. They should be lightened, and shaped and brushed to as much of an arch as possible. To lighten the eyebrows you can bleach them with a cream bleach. The bleaches that are especially designed for facial hair work well. But, this is a job that should only be done at a beauty salon; or if you want to do it at home get the help of a friend and be very sure your eyes are closed and well protected during the carefully-timed bleaching.

If you want to see the effect of lighter brows, you can brush a lighter color into the brows. This is done by brushing your eyebrows against the eyebrow crayon and then brushing the picked up color on the hair of the brows. You can easily and safely go from black brows to dark brown, or from brown to light brown in this way.

EYEGLASSES

Just because you wear glasses doesn't mean you should look dowdy. Quite the contrary, glasses give you one more opportunity to look your best. You can choose from an endless variety of eye- and face-framing eyeglass frames.

Colors and shapes vary with fashion, but within any fashion there are basic rules in selecting the color, weight, and shape best for you.

If you have a *round* face with full cheeks and round, large eyes, select a square frame that will not repeat the curves of your round face. If you have a low forehead, keep the nose bridge low, about halfway between the frames.

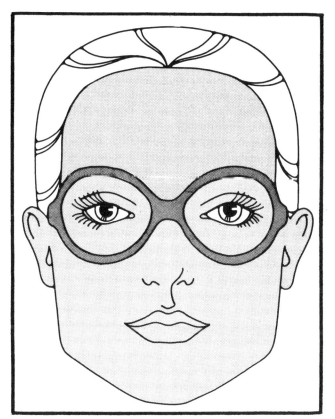

Round Frames

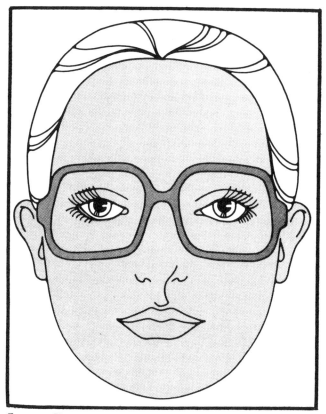

Square Frames

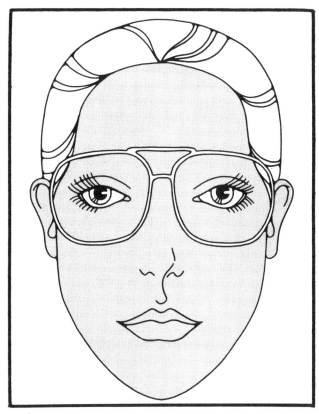

Delicate Frames

If you have a *square jaw* or a *triangular-shaped* face with a pointed chin, select rounded oval frames that will draw attention to your temples rather than the lower part of your face. A small metallic ornament on the glasses, or contrasting color earpieces, will do this.

A *narrow face,* or an oval face with a high forehead, should have delicate frames that hold large or deep lenses. The nose bridge should be fairly high and the glasses should seem to wrap around your face.

If you have small, delicate features and a narrow neck and body, you'll probably look best in thin, lightweight frames that are close in color to your own hair. But if you have large features, such as a long nose, large protruding eyes, and thick lips, select frames that combine straight and rounded shapes. The top of the frames should cover your brows and an intense but muted color might be very attractive.

THE NOSE

According to the ideal proportions of classical sculpture, the nose—the most conspicuous but seldom discussed feature—should be one-third of the entire length of the face. The space between the eyes at the bridge of the nose should be exactly the same width as an eye, and this should also equal the measurement at the widest point of the nostrils.

According to this same ideal, the length of the nose should equal the length of the ear. It should also equal the distance between the tip of the nose and the bottom of the chin.

The nose juts out from the plane of the cheeks and forehead, and the angle at which it meets the face is very important to the appearance. If the nose were flat, it would be 180°; if it were at right angles, it would be 90°. The attractiveness of any nose depends on the length of the nose and the shape of the nostrils and forehead.

The nose should also tilt slightly upward at the tip. The angle at which the nose and the upper lip meet should be slightly upward—more than 90°.

A "nose bob," cosmetic surgery to change the size, tilt, or shape of the nose, is one of the most sought-after procedures. If you should go to a plastic surgeon, he will probably make all sorts of judgments about the angles and proportions of your nose.

One of the most common beauty problems is a bump or hump in the nose (although in ancient Roman times a hump was considered a sign of beauty and high status). A large nose, a hooked nose with the end dropping down, and a long nose are also considered less than attractive. These problems are corrected by using a combination of darker than normal and lighter than normal foundation colors, or by carefully applying blusher or shadow.

Very often the nose is just too wide or the nostrils too thick. Sometimes, when the upper lip is too short or the nostrils are too close together or too far apart, the entire nose just seems out of proportion even though in theory the nose is ideal for your face shape.

Look at the nose charts; each shows a small picture of a profile of a nose and next to it a description of the nose.

Then, trace the full-sized nose, do your best to make it similar to your own nose, or try at least to lengthen or shorten it to show some of the basic configurations of your nose. Measure the width across the tip of your nose and nostrils. Adjust the nose sample to reflect the width of your nose. The length of the sample must also be adjusted to reflect the length of your own nose.

Here are the most common complaints and directions for improving the appearance of your nose, improving its proportion so that it suits your face, and camouflaging or obscuring the less-than-perfect aspects of the nose. The same principle holds: using dark to diminish and applying light, or reflective, to make some sections appear more prominent. For daytime sculpturing, use a blended foundation—one dark shade and one shade lighter with a tiny blend of rouge for a slightly sun-kissed look. For nighttime, a white highlight and a dab of reflective silver or gold sparklers to catch the light might be best. In day or night avoid too-white or too deep shadings; and, of course, blend well!

1 *Short with a bump at the bridge* Apply dark over the bump; lengthen the nose with light at the top and bottom of nostrils.
2 *Long with a bump at the bridge* Darken over the bump; shorten the nose with a dark tip and dark on the bridge between the nostrils.
3 *Too long from bridge to nostrils* Shorten at bridge by darkening from point even with bottom lid to brows; darken tip and shorten with dab of rouge under nostrils.
4 *Long at tip* Lift by applying light on tip to mid-bridge; put slightly darkened shade on nostrils.
5 *Thick throughout* Slightly shade down the sides of the nose; leave a straight unshaded line down the center of the nose.
6 *Thick, lumpy nostrils* If pores are enlarged, use astringent before applying makeup. Gently dab a darker shade of foundation on sides of nostrils; draw attention away from nose with dramatic eye makeup.
7 *Large nostrils* Be sure nostrils are free of hair. Use wax on open portions of nostrils, or just a dab of hair depilatory may work. If you use a chemical depilatory, no more than a movement or two should be enough; the skin is very sensitive and the pores tend to enlarge easily. If the nostrils are well shaped and even, then the job is to direct attention to another part of the face. Do this with an application of lighter than skin tone cover or foundation to the upper nose. Pat and press makeup from bridge over to the inner eye, on the sides of the nose only.
8 *Bulbous nose* This must be approached very deftly. It will require a bit of practice not to have a dirty nose effect. Very lightly cover the end of the nose with a slightly darker shade

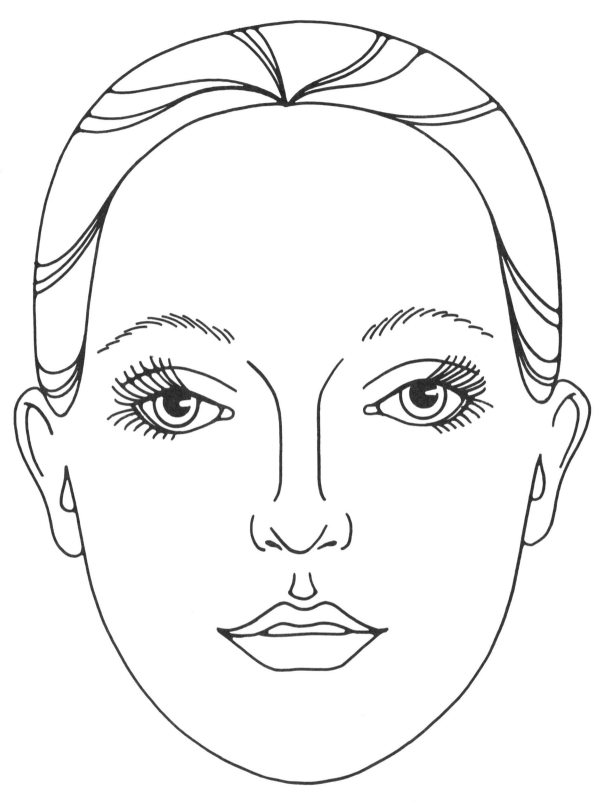

Perfect Nose—Front

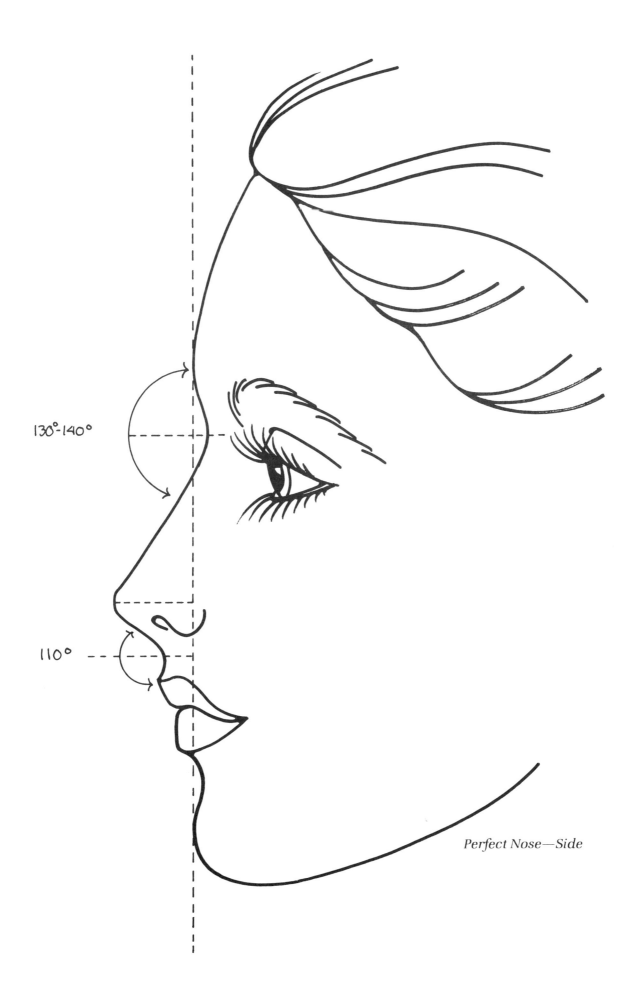

130°-140°

110°

Perfect Nose—Side

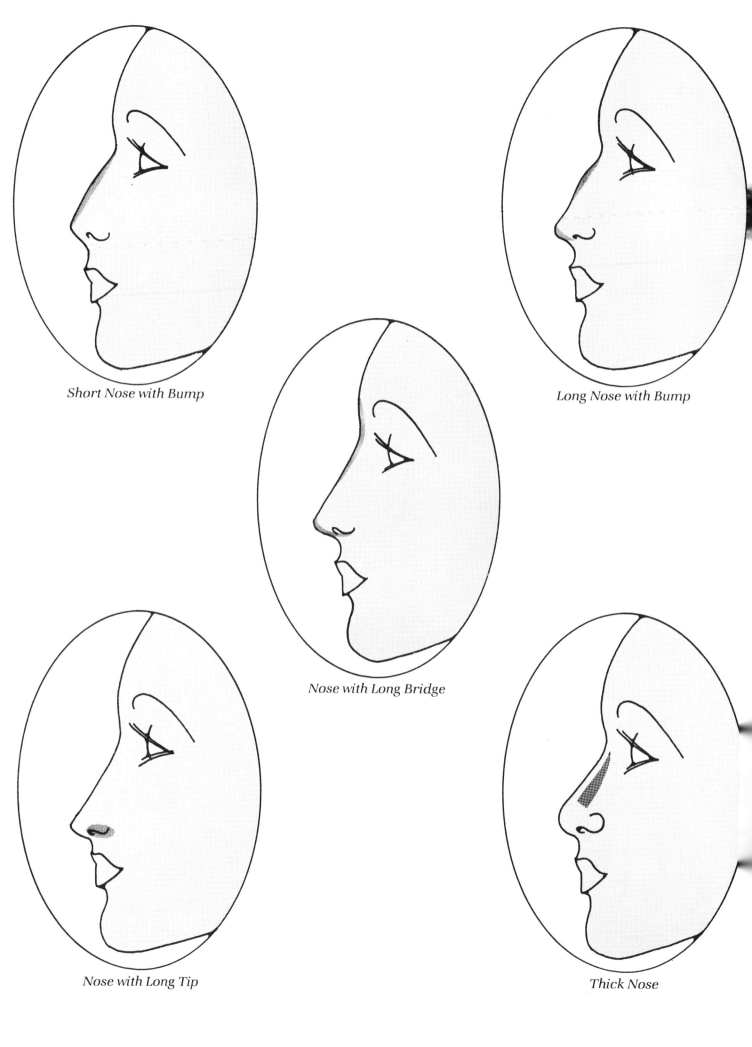

Short Nose with Bump

Long Nose with Bump

Nose with Long Bridge

Nose with Long Tip

Thick Nose

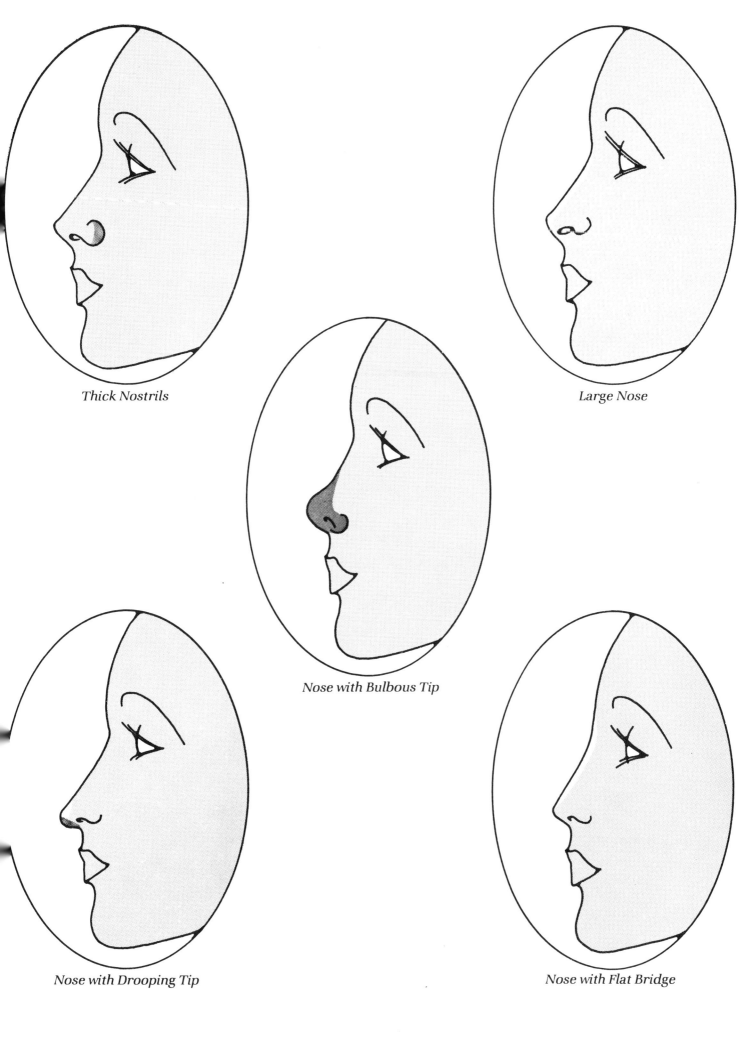

Thick Nostrils

Large Nose

Nose with Bulbous Tip

Nose with Drooping Tip

Nose with Flat Bridge

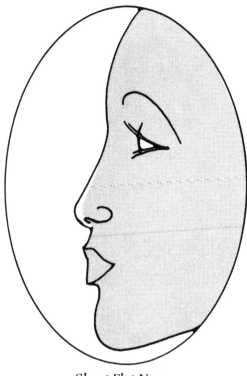

Short Flat Nose

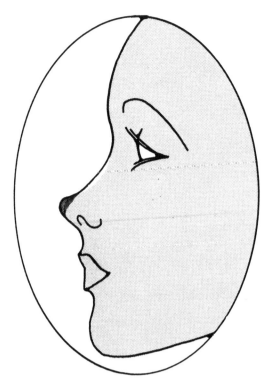

Pug Nose

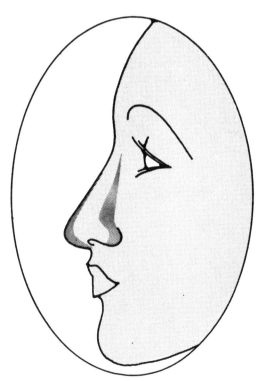

Long Broad Nose

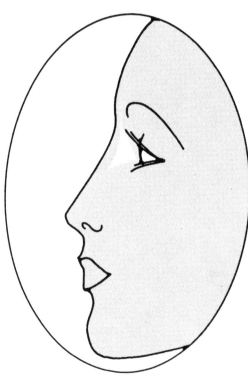

Nose with High Bridge

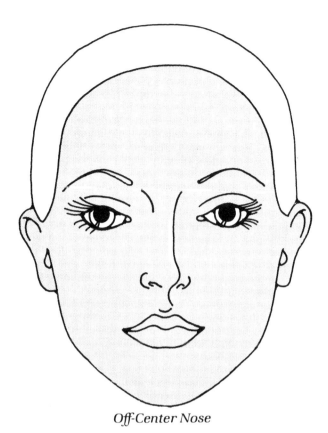

Off-Center Nose

Uneven Nostrils

of foundation and blend with the normal shade upward toward the bridge and down on the sides.

9 *Drooping tip* To raise the nose visually, put a tiny dot of light color at the very center of the top end, just at the point where the nose turns under toward the nostrils. The underside of the nose should be darkened slightly.

10 *Flat at the bridge* A streak of light color about one-quarter of an inch wide should be positioned on the very top of the nose from bridge to tip. Shade to a point at the tip.

11 *Short and flat* Put a streak of light color down the top center of the nose, over the tip and over the strip between the nostrils and the bottom of the nose.

12 *Pug nose* The ski-jump nose is great for comedy, but not very glamorous or elegant. The top of the tip should be darkened, and the area just before the tip slightly lightened.

13 *Long and broad* Shorten with dark shading on bottom, and narrow with delicate shading on the sides.

14 *High, narrow bridge* Widen the bridge area by applying a light color to the sides of the upper nose, and blend the light color up to the inner corner of each eye and upward to the eyebrow. Do not allow the light color to cover the top of the bridge.

15 *Nose off-center* If the nose is slightly to the right, use lighter color on the right side than on the left; if it is slightly to the left, then put the lighter color to the plane of the left side and a slightly darker to the right.

16 *Uneven nostrils* The larger should be shadowed slightly, to be just a bit darker.

LIPS

Lips are a focal point of any face. Your lips are probably the balance counterpoint to your eyes. Of the five pairs of lips illustrated select the lips most like your own and position them under your plastic Beauty Palette. After the lips are positioned, use a lip pencil, a crayon, or a china marking pencil to trace your lip shape. You can use almost any type of lip color, just as there are a variety of lip colors available for your own lips.

Next to each pair of lips is a suggestion for perfecting your lip-look. The following are also some lip ideas that can be adapted to your own mouth.

1 Find out how your lips fit the basic proportions of your face. Your nose should be about one-third of your face, and from the bottom of the nose to tip of the chin should be another one-third. That means the distance between your nose and lips shouldn't be too long or too short.
2 Thin lips seem fuller with a bright lipstick.
3 Lips seem fuller if the outer edges are darker than the middle.
4 The tops of the curves of your upper lip look best when they are directly under the center of each nostril. Move the curve slightly if you need to. If the color disappears almost as soon as you apply your lipstick, you probably need to use a foundation under it.
5 Make a smiling mouth by turning the outer edges of your lip up slightly. It makes for a younger look.
6 An overextended or heavy upper lip will give you a sneering expression.
7 Don't suck your teeth or purse or pucker your lips; it will give you an old-looking, withered mouth.
8 Clenching your jaws can give you an ugly, sharp line at the lips, and also a

muscle tension headache. (Clenching your teeth can also do permanent damage to your teeth and jaw.)
9 A large lower lip needs a darker upper lip than lower lip.
10 Your lips should look as pretty in speech as in repose; make sure your lips move gracefully in action.
11 Singing is good exercise for your lips. Another good exercise is to master tongue twisters. Use "p" and "m" sounds; they stretch the muscle around the mouth.

Even, Full Lips Avoid the deepest colors that contrast greatly with the skin. A receding or weak chin can be overpowered by full lips (Liza Minnelli), but drawing the lower lip smaller than the natural line and adding white to the chin will refocus the visual proportions.

Even curves can be minimized, and a too-full mouth reduced by painting the shape slightly within the natural lip line. Muted shades, similar to the inner lip and gums, might also diminish the too-heavy look. Counter thickness by extending the sides.

Lips Out of Proportion Use a darker shade of lipstick and a heavy lip gloss on the uneven section of your lip. The lower right of these lips can be made fuller just through darker colorings. If you lack a cupid's bow, you can draw one in.

Uneven Shape, Uneven Color A pale green undercoat moisturizer or a skin-tone coverstick can be used to blank out the lip shape and color before shaping with lip-

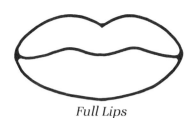

Full Lips

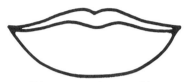

Disproportionate Lips

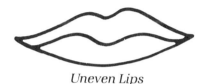

Uneven Lips

Thin Lips

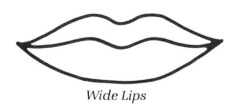

Wide Lips

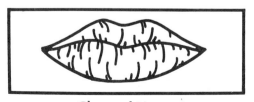

Chapped Lips

stick. Try to match the two lips so both upper and lower are of equal width and length.

Thin Lips Thin or small lips can wear a deep color. But avoid the bright slash of color for a thin mouth shape. Use gloss and a lighter color in the center for high lights. Paint in fullness by using darker colors on the sides.

Wide Lips Well-shaped wide lips can be an asset; as an example notice Cheryl Tiegs' firm and beautiful mouth. But, if you feel that your mouth is just too wide for the sides of your face and overpowers your jaw, you can make your lips look narrower by using a dark lipcolor and lots of gloss in the center of the mouth. Do not paint the outer edges of the lips.

Lip laments are many. Here is a list of the most common and some of the solutions:

Chapped Lips Come winter, use a moisturizer under your lip color, a gloss over the color. Resist any urge to lick your lips; you'll be licking away the protective gloss.

Cracked and Wrinkled Lips This might indicate poor general health. Watch your diet. Are you getting enough foods rich in vitamin B_2? This vitamin is in liver and cooked leafy vegetables.

Blistex is a medicated lip conditioner-moisturizer that keeps your lips smooth and healthy.

Brigitte Bardot, the famous French beauty and movie star, always has a box full of Blistex with her when she travels.

Sunburned Lips Some lip gloss contains sunblock. Check the labels before you buy.

Herpes Virus This virus can cause small sores that resist healing. It should be treated by a doctor.

Bleeding, Fuzzy, and Feathering Lipstick This condition could mean your lipstick is too greasy or that you need to use a lip pencil to outline your lips.

Color Changes You haven't found the lip color that is most suitable for your body chemistry. A tinted moisturizer (see moisturizers) on your foundation might serve as a primer coat.

Color Washout You are not applying your lip color correctly. Try using the following technique:

1 Apply a concealer stick or a creme foundation.
2 Outline the lips with a pencil, or with a lip brush if you prefer to use a brush.
3 Apply powder.
4 Blot by pressing a tissue against the lips.
5 Apply a thin coat of lip color, then gloss, and over the gloss apply another coat of lip color.

Lipsticks and lip colorings are the most popular of any skin coloring. Lipsticks became part of makeup after World War I, and even during the great Depression of the Thirties women refused to give up their metal-cased color stick. Recent years have brought endless variety in types of containers, texture, and viscosity, and even color.

The basic stick of pigment in a waxy crayon is ever popular. Transparent colors can come in sticks or tiny jars; they have more lubricants and provide a shinier surface than the stick, but less color. Transparent and semi-transparent lipsticks provide a glossy, slick overcoat with a soft, glowing shine like stained glass. Glosses, polishes, gels, and shiners, some clear and some with tints, are transparent colors. The most recent are viscous and put on with small sponge wands, or flavored for taste and rolled on. Frosted lip colors—both lipsticks and glosses—have luminescent, pearly shades and light reflectors right in the formulas.

TEETH

Lips can be attractive only if the teeth beneath the lips are strong, clean, and sparkling. The teeth must be in firm gums, and there should be a good foundation of bones.

The relative fullness and some of the actual shape of your lips are partly dependent on the position of the teeth. It is almost impossible for you to get your lipstick on correctly and neatly and for the shape to be even, if you are missing a tooth or if your mouth has any tender or sore spots.

When your teeth, gums, and mouth are not properly cleaned after eating, small bits of food stick to the sides of the teeth. The material decays and breeds masses of germ life, commonly called "plaques." Sensitive, bleeding gums are a sign of trouble. No technique, lip brush, color, or special gloss can make up for a decayed tooth. And certainly the foul breath that is part of the infection that caused the decay is the enemy of beauty.

Plaques are difficult to see because they take on the coloration of the healthy tissue, but they can easily be seen if they are stained with special dyes. There are some commercial dyes that you can find at the drug store, but green food coloring is just as good. It can be bought in any grocery store or supermarket and a small cotton swab is all you need. Dip the cotton swab in the jar of coloring and brush the bright green color across the top of your teeth on the gum line, and into the cracks between the teeth. The plaque will take the stain so you can see just where it is hiding. With a very soft toothbrush (this is the one time that nylon is better than natural bristles) brush away all the stained material. Rinse and brush again until it is all gone.

Another way of clearing bacterial deposits from tooth surfaces is to floss your teeth every time you eat. Here is the correct way to floss:

1 Use about 18 inches of unwaxed floss, or dental tape.
2 Hold the floss between your thumb and two fingers of each hand. This will give you control of the floss movement. Pull the floss entirely through the small cracks between the teeth. Work back and forth several times.
3 Don't skip any teeth. Work on the front teeth as well as the sides and back. Some teeth will require several flossings.
4 For the bottom row hold the floss between the two fingers and thumbs as before, and push with a strong downward motion. Try not to pull the lips out of shape unnecessarily.
5 After flossing each crevice, pull the floss all the way through the hole, dropping one end of the floss. Never try to pull the floss from the gums to the edge of the teeth; it will weaken fillings and caps.
6 Rinse the mouth after flossing every few teeth to rid your mouth of the nasty debris that you have loosened from your teeth and gums.

After flossing, brush your teeth well to keep them smooth and polished. When brushing, don't forget a final brushing of the tongue.

Avoid between-meal snacks. The fewer food contacts you have, the less chance plaque has to form: bacteria live on the food residue. Try not to eat, drink, suck, or chew any gum or liquid that might have sugar in it; this includes alcoholic beverages. Good teeth care will keep you on a good total diet. The actress Angie Dickinson, noted for her beautiful figure and sparkling smile, claims that she diets by brushing her teeth every time she has an urge to eat a food that is not part of her program. The brushing takes up a few minutes, and it keeps her mouth sparkling clean and fresh as well as helping to resist a no-no for both her mouth and figure.

HAIR

Around your perfect face, your hair should be a frame that shows all of your features to their best advantage and creates a background for your total look. Like your features, the frame must be in proportion. It must be the right color (blonde, brownette, black) and the right texture (straight, wavy, curling) to show your nose, eyes, and lips to the best advantage—and in some cases your hair should be styled to show your neck and ears as part of your facial features.

A famous television actress rose to popularity on the strength of her bouncy blonde hair, and there are countless movie and TV stars, models, and actresses who are known for their beautiful hair. Like other parts of the body, the hair must be immaculately clean to be beautiful.

Shampoo is probably the basis of all hair treatment. Before the late 1930's almost all shampoos were made of a formulation of soap. Since that time, synthetic cleaners and detergents have been added to the soap with varying results. Soap, an alkali of salt and fatty acids, works well in removing dirt and grease from surfaces of the skin and hair, but in water that contains calcium (hard water), soap reacts with the calcium and forms soap scum, that nasty residue that causes bathtub rings. Synthetics don't form soap scum, but they can cause severe eye irritation, and many people are allergic to some of the substances in synthetic detergents. If there is any irritation of your scalp, or if your hair really feels awful after shampooing, you might want to try a pure soap shampoo, such as a castile shampoo or even a cake of soap, and then rinse your hair with vinegar, lemon, or some other acid solution that will get rid of the alkali scum.

Detergent shampoos labeled for use on normal, dry, or oily hair are formulated by controlling the strength of the synthetic detergent, whose ability to strip dirt and oil from the hair is noted by those labels. How a shampoo looks—its viscosity, clarity or creaminess, color, or smell—has little to do with its ability to clean the hair and still leave the strands undamaged. A medicated shampoo, designed to rid the scalp of small flakes of dead skin, can be just as gentle as a baby shampoo.

If you are unhappy with the texture of your hair—if it doesn't have body, hold a set or is fly-away—this can be due to the quality of the atmosphere as much as to your hair texture. The glamorous Diane von Fürstenberg claims she avoided trips to Brazil for fear the damp climate would make her hair unmanageable.

Your Hairline After perfecting your features, you should now consider again how the shape of your forehead affects the proportions of your face and how well your features fit your face. Notice your hairline: Is it even? Is it a clear, distinct line, or fuzzy? Does your hair look best over your forehead or pulled away? If the line is fuzzy, and it bothers you, you can easily have it cleaned to a smooth neat line, or a new shape, by electrolysis. Cher, as well as many another famous face, has had her hairline re-drawn.

Most faces look best with a casual, relaxed hairdo. Unless your features are perfect, you should not attempt a slicked-back smooth hairline. A soft hairline is most attractive with an older face. Be sure that the hair near your temples is clean, and not covered with makeup. Clean away the extra makeup with a soft swab of cotton. Do not use alcohol or oil: alcohol will dry your hair and oil will have a greasy residue.

Always pin your hair back or cover it with a shower cap before washing your face; wash it carefully and be sure to rinse every bit of residue of soap from the hairline.

Flattery for Grey Hair

It can be silvery and sparkling; it can frame and lighten your face and actually make your skin seem lustrous. Or, it can be dingy, dirty, and depressing. Blondes and redheads usually find less alteration in their coloring than women who had dark hair. Black women will notice the most dramatic change. Their dark skin highlighted with a silverish halo can make their eyes look more vibrant and alive.

If your hair is grey, you might select lipsticks that reflect pleasantly on the color of your teeth. If your teeth are yellowish or have any stains, avoid a lipstick that contains any orange or yellowish color. Try rosy pinks, but avoid any lipstick that is too bluish, because it will make your gums look bruised and purplish.

Dark eyebrows can be overpowering with grey hair. Consider lightening your brows with bleach or tweezing them so that they are slightly thinner than they were. If your brows are turning grey, you might want to even out the color with bleach or by brushing with eye shadow.

Grey hair is often wiry and seems to curl without much grace. But there is no need to wear a bun just because your hair is grey; there is nothing so attractive as grey or silver hair in a loose-flowing style. Softness of style is particularly flattering to a mature face.

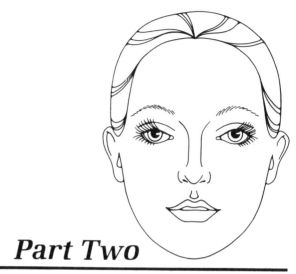

Part Two

MAKEOVERS

WHY A MAKEOVER?

At age 28, Tina found herself a widow with three small children. Coming home from her lawyer's office about two months after her husband's funeral, she caught sight of herself in a store mirror. She was shocked: she still looks like a teenager, and the slight sprinkle of freckles across her nose doesn't help to convince anyone—even Tina—that she is a responsible adult.

Marjorie married late. Now at 60, after twelve years of marriage, she is facing divorce. She feels she has hardly lived and wants a new and exciting life.

Ethel needs at least $30,000 a year to enjoy life. As a young and very beautiful woman, she receives a great deal of attention and has grown used to exclusive restaurants and a luxurious life style. She is exhilarated by meeting successful and famous men, and although she is now a secretary in a large midwestern stockbroker's office, she plans to become a partner—within only a few years.

Anne, putting on her daughter's crown for a school play, saw herself in the reflected mirrors on the crown. She decided it was time for a makeover.

Jean's two sons are in college. She's taken a job as a secretary in a small construction firm and finds that the nicest part of her job is getting out of the office and into the open air. She is considering—at 37—becoming a carpenter.

There are many reasons for changing one's appearance: growth, challenges, new options, and just feeling good about yourself. Most people are honest. When they look like someone else, they feel somehow dishonest. A makeover is designed to present you—but you at your very best.

FINDING YOUR OWN SPECIAL LOOK

If you had to meet someone who didn't know you, how would you describe yourself? Don't be modest . . . truthfully, if you have good features you should work *with* them.

Are You the Teen Type?

Are you between 14 and 19 years of age, with a small quick figure? Do you wear junior sizes? Would you like to be seen on the pages of *Seventeen?* The teen type is often described as cute, fresh, innocent, vivacious, happy, and often full of great energy. Your skin might have a tendency to be oily, and an occasional blemish may be a source of distress. Even if you are a dark brunette or black, your skin is bright and lively, and you can wear very dramatic makeup. But you probably look best keeping your looks wholesome and natural. You don't get dressed up too often, so probably your grooming tips must be related to your everyday school look. You'll find the right makeover program for your special beauty in the first section of each of the skin-tone charts.

Are You a Dramatic High-fashion Model Type?

Are you between the ages of 17 and 24, and might you look even a bit older when wearing glamorous clothing? Are you slender and in good health? Can you wear high-fashion and very extreme clothing? Do you follow the latest styles and often experiment with new colors of makeup? Your type might be found in the pages of *Glamour* or *Vogue*. You are probably just starting a career, or perhaps you are in college. It is important for you to give the right impression on job interviews, and you might also find yourself invited to special parties and other dress-up occasions. You'll want to look your best—but not overdone or "cheap looking."

Are You a Sophisticated Type?

Are you between 22 and about 30 years of age, and just making the first steps advancing in your career, or meeting some of the people who can make a difference in your future? If so, you'll want to give the right impression at all times. If you have a pretty face, play it up—your skin and figure are probably at their best, and even if you are an outdoor girl, you are wise enough to guard against the aging effects of sun, wind, and pollution. If you work in a large city, you'll have to be especially careful of industrial

pollution and the drying effects of air-conditioning. You'll probably be going back home frequently, getting together with old friends or going to high school reunions. You'll want a complete makeover to look your best.

Are You a Young Housewife/Mother?

Are you between 19 and 30, with one or two children under the age of seven, and do you do more than eight loads of washing every week? Do you often feel that you just don't have a moment for yourself? You're right. This is a busy time in your life, and it's easy to fall into bad habits of neglecting grooming. But, although you are rushed, you have a friendly, wholesome, happy, and pleasant disposition, and except for periods of slight depression, life seems full of excitement. You might be found in the pages of *Woman's Day*, *Family Circle*, or *Glamour* magazine. You would like to hold a full-time job, and if you don't, you are conscious of financial pressure as well as the time pressures that your present responsibilities put on you.

Are You a Woman In Your Prime—Your Thirties and Forties?

Are you between 28 and about 42 and enjoying the most active and vital period of your life? Are you looking for a way of projecting yourself, of showing the "real you"? You might wear size 6 or 16, but you are mature, and you want to project a competent, pleasant, and happy vision of yourself. You might be seen in the pages of *McCall's* or *Ladies' Home Journal.* You may notice that you've been gaining weight slowly, and it seems more difficult than it used to be to take it off. You're looking forward to your college or high school anniversary . . . and you're wondering what happened to the pretty girl who once could wear anything and look fine. You have to dress with a bit more care now.

Are You a Mature and Elegant Woman?

Are you over 40 and probably over 50, whether plump or still youthfully slender? Have you noticed that your skin isn't as taut as it used to be, and there are dry lines around your eyes and perhaps some softness under your chin? Some people might call you "motherly"—but you are really ready for a whole new life. Many people admire you, and you have many satisfactions in seeing those about you grow and develop, but you want to look your very best and to be as attractive as possible as a woman. You're very concerned about the effects of menopause on your skin and on your looks in general. Your hair has some grey in it, and your beauty techniques and beauty program need some updating so that you don't seem dowdy.

Do You Have a Special Kind of Beauty?

Are you dark-skinned and do you trace your ancestors to South America or to Africa? Have you managed to work out your own individual beauty program to emphasize your special qualities? You must deal with some annoying beauty problems—such as "ashy skin" that requires constant care, and hair that tends to break easily and to be a bit dry. But happily, your skin is still glassy soft and resilient. And no one really dare guess your age—if you get enough rest and take good care of yourself. If you have a tendency to put on weight, you must be on a careful diet at all times. You and your husband or some special friend might be getting ready for a wonderful vacation, or you might be going to a family reunion, and you'll want to look your best.

TAKING A GOOD LOOK: How to Look at Yourself

Now that you've found your look, let's see how to attain it. You must begin with a careful, honest study of your features. But how?

We see reflections of ourselves in small bathroom mirrors, or fleetingly in store windows, but when do we really see ourselves the way others see us? Very seldom. To do a makeover, you must see clearly what you are making over.

First, you need to see yourself in a good light. The lighting near your mirror should be as close as possible to natural light. Use a mirror area that has the light coming from behind you.

Second, get a good mirror. A

mirror's quality can be checked by moving toward and away from it and seeing if there is any distortion in your reflection. Pay special attention to the top and bottom of a full-length mirror.

Next, don't stand in one position straight-on to your mirror. You are seldom seen from that direct position. Move in front of the mirror. See how you look bending, reaching, and shaking. If you usually wear glasses, be sure you use them when examining your own reflection in the mirror.

Now what do you look like? Study your best points first: don't start out being too critical. If you have nice shoulders, or a pert nose, notice that feature first.

Now smile at yourself. Your smile is your most important beauty aid. No matter how perfect your makeup is, your real makeover will be in your feeling about yourself that you automatically convey to others.

THE MAKEUP INVENTORY

You've probably read many articles that describe the perfect tool for makeup application. Most makeup artists use a combination of brushes and sponges. These are satisfactory for the professionals because they are working on another person's face. But these tools are difficult for many people to use on themselves; they find the tension or pressure of the brush is uneven. I've never been able to feel as con-fident, or get as satisfying effects, as I can with just my fingers. I know just how hard to press; and if my fingers are feeling a bit stiff, as they do on an occasional morning, I can still manage, although I could never do so with several brushes to juggle. Even powder and rouge seem to go on best with just a fingertip.

Another reason I use my fingers is that I'm lazy. I don't want to spend ten minutes cleaning the brushes after I use them, and if the brushes are not cleaned, I feel that they gather gunk and bacteria.

There are two exceptions: eye makeup and lip makeup. With both, a sharp pencil can be mastered easily, and pencils can be kept very clean by sharpening just before use. But don't waste money on tools that you cannot use or that make upkeep difficult.

Using a combination of skin covers and powder, creme or stick colors, you can create endless effects. But before you go out and buy anything, be guided by some very simple rules: First, buy the smallest size, *always*. Second, if you don't like the effect, or if it is unpleasant or difficult to handle, or if you even slightly suspect the product of being irritating—throw it out. *Out*, as fast as possible, so you won't be even slightly tempted to use it, and so it doesn't just sit around gathering dust.

In a hardware store or at a notions counter, buy a flat, unframed mirror. This mirror will serve as your table. It will reflect your face from underneath and act as a reflector for the light that you use to provide for your makeover. Try to position your makeup area near a window. If you make up in the bathroom, as many people do, use incandescent lights. Position a 60-watt bulb on the upper right and upper left of the mirror. Your flat mirror should be set in the middle of a large tray so that you can balance it over the sink bowl as you make up, and then carry it away when you no longer need it.

Your Makeup Inventory Should Include:

1 small bottle of vegetable oil (the smallest size olive oil does well)
1 small bottle of baby oil, to remove makeup
2 glass jars with spray pumps, for spraying face with mineral water
small sterile gauze pads, for applying liquids and evening powder
sterile cotton balls
white paper napkins (they really are more absorbent than tissues)
1 small jar of moisturizer
1 small jar of Vaseline
1 box of toothpicks for mixing makeup and making cotton-tipped tools
1 small hand pencil sharpener
1 eyebrow brush

Coloring

1 liquid, lighter in shade than skin tone, water soluble
1 creme or cake makeup, a shade darker than your own
1 white cover creme
2 colors shadow darker than skin: brown, grey, green, etc., or any combintion

Powders

2 shades lighter than skin, pearlized or frosted, white, sand-beige, or dove grey
1 blusher powder for oily skin, creme for dry skin, powder for oily or normal complexions
2 wands of mascara, one darker than the other (a great combination is dark brown and wine)
2 eyebrow pencils: one brown, one charcoal grey or black
2 red-tone lip pencils (red and wine-pink are good)
1 deep lip color or transparent stain gel, pot or stick
1 frosted lip color, pot or stick
1 jar of vitamin E capsules, for nourishing mask for dry skin around the eye area
1 bottle aspirin, which contain salicylic acid; two tablets, moistened and crushed in the palm, make a good exfoliating mask, and a soothing antiseptic, for oily skin

HOW TO USE YOUR MAKEOVER CHART

The following pages are devoted to helping you plan your own makeover. You've now had a chance to experiment, to create various effects with makeup in order to achieve the look you want. The charts have been developed to enable you to create the effect you want, according to the type you are or want to be, consistent with your own coloring and your own age or peer group, whether for morning, business, or a gala evening.

I've used the word "brownette" to describe the pale-skinned, brown-haired type that is so common.

This type is not blonde. She sometimes has lighter skin than a blonde, but she often has reddish to dark brown hair. The skin tone and the makeup are entirely different from those of a true brunette, who is an olive-skinned, or even ivory-skinned, woman with black hair and dark brows and lashes. If you are a light to medium ash-brown blonde, you may want to look up both "brownette" and "blonde." Similarly, if you have a dark complexion, you can look up both brownette and brunette.

Who are you? What is your age? What sort of clothing will you be wearing? What colors are your favorites? All of these elements are charted on the makeover charts. You'll notice that the charts are divided into "time of day" or "occasions," so that you will know exactly what sort of makeover is right for each situation. There is also a section of Special Notes, as well as information about jewelry or accessories that will highlight your makeover. Sandwiched in are other tips and bits of advice in answer to questions that might come up as you use the charts.

You will notice that the popular color blue is seldom suggested for eye shadow or liner; try something new, such as berry, brown, rust, or taupe. You'll find these so much more flattering, so much more natural, and so much newer. We've tried to focus on the latest shades of makeup that are popular in Europe and the United States.

Now you are ready to proceed with your makeover. First find your "role-model" celebrity, and then look at the chart that shows a face. Copy the colors and shades that are for you, for your makeover, and in that way keep a complete record of makeovers for reference. It is also fun to suggest a makeover for a close friend, or even plan how you would make over your favorite movie star for a special role. You can become your own makeup artist.

YOUR MAKEOVER

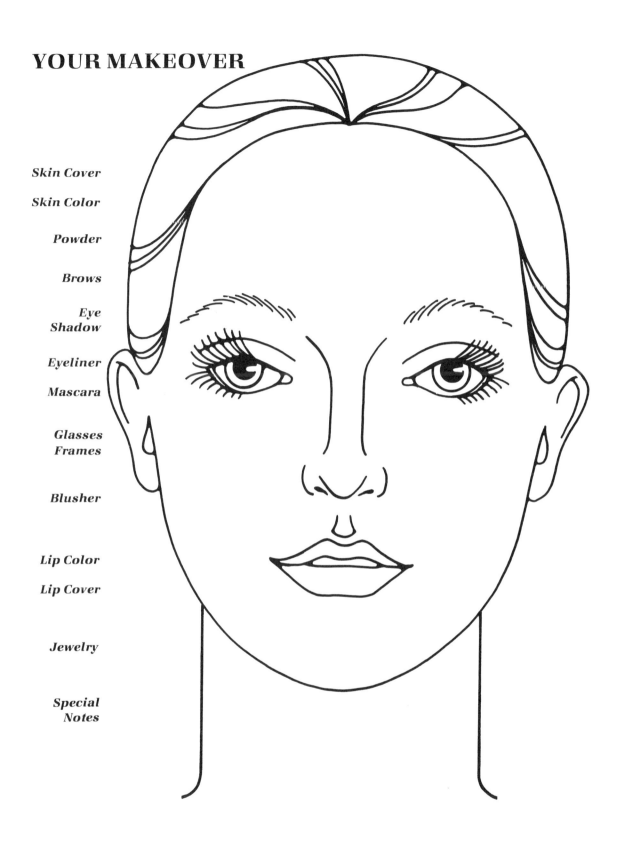

Skin Cover

Skin Color

Powder

Brows

Eye
Shadow

Eyeliner

Mascara

Glasses
Frames

Blusher

Lip Color

Lip Cover

Jewelry

Special
Notes

WORKING BLONDE

Suzanne Somers, Cheryl Tiegs, Cheryl Ladd, Candice Bergen,
Farrah Fawcett-Majors, Lindsay Wagner

	Morning/Sports	School/Work/Home	Evening/Parties
Skin Cover	Moisturizer/ sun screen.	Moisturizer, coverstick.	Moisturizer, coverstick.
Skin Color	No.	Beige, rose. Use a light, thin coat; don't attempt to cover all blemishes.	Excitement can make your face flush. Use ivory, peach, yellow.
Powder	No.	Cream red rose, cinnamon, and titians.	Ambers, honey, roses, pinks, lavender (with pink lipstick).
Brows	Brushed and shaped, they can be professionally dyed honey brown to deep brown; keep brows one shade lighter than your hair.	Fill in sparse hairs with a brow-brush that has been brushed against beige charcoal, or use brown pencil.	Grey, brown.
Eye Shadow	Sage, muted grey-browns, grey-greens.	Cinnamons, pumpkins, beiges, browns; gold-green highlights.	Violet, plum, wine, beige, grey; white-pearl for brow bone.
Eyeliner	Smudged gently; a natural color.	Carefully applied, dotted with sable brush; greys, deep nut-browns, fawns.	Greys, browns, deep violets.
Mascara	Heavy coat in brown or grey.	Browns, greys, and wine.	Browns, greys, soft blacks.
Glasses Frames	Sunglasses should be used for all outdoor activities. Grey and green lenses are most soothing to the eyes; blue and yellow actually can intensify a glare.	Match to hair color.	Pink, white, frameless.
Lip Color	Rosy pinks; almost any color except bright red.	Gentle reds, clear plums, and berry colors should define the lips.	Corals, oranges, golden reds, sparkling wines.
Lip Cover	Transparent gloss.	Heavy gloss will make your lips look fuller, and also protect them.	A dab of gold-metallic eye sha-dow in the center of your lip will catch the light in evening wear.
Blusher	Pinked beiges, corals, peach colors.	Avoid a painted or blotchy look by blending blusher with your foundation.	Intense color (not dark color) will prevent an evening wash-out look.
Special Notes	Think Cheryl Tiegs: healthy, sun-drenched, vital. But be sure you use a sun guard and avoid sunburn.	Brown-eyed blondes should play up their eyes with dark brown liner and using heavy mascara.	A child's toothbrush makes a good brush for brows, and keeping makeup off your hair-line. Never brush wet hair.
Jewelry	Sports watches with black rub-berized bands are attractive and useful.	Gold chains look classic and elegant. Do not match jewelry, except in shades and feeling. Keep stones or pins matched to eye color.	Use your hair as jewelry. Twine it with beads, metallics, ribbons.

TEEN BLONDE
Jody Foster, Sally Struthers

	Morning/Sports	School/Work/Home	Evening/Parties
Skin Cover	Wash nose, chin, and forehead often. Cover eye area with a moisturizer, even if you are in your early teens.	Cover eye area with moisturizer. Neck and shoulders are sensitive, too.	Moisturizer on entire face.
Skin Color	No.	Water-soluble liquid makeup on nose, chin, and forehead.	Liquid foundation in ivory, bisque, or beige.
Powder	No.	No.	No.
Brows	Tweeze only stray hairs between brows.	Tweeze only stray hairs between brows. Pencil in missing or sparse areas on brows with light brown pencil.	Tweeze center section to directly over inner eye.
Eye Shadow	No.	No.	Brown, gold, honey, oak, and silver to pewter grey accent your light eyes.
Eyeliner	No.	Light brown, liquid dot of lashes.	No, unless your lashes are very light.
Mascara	Light to medium.	Tawny to medium brown coat of mascara.	No.
Glasses Frames	Match to hair color or try frames of light brown, amber, or pink.	Match to hair color, or try frames of light brown, amber, or pink.	Silver or gold wire frames.
Lip Color	Pink, peach lip stain only.	Apply transparent gloss-stain from pots with finger or use gloss from tubes.	Rose, pink, melon, and plum.
Lip Cover	Gloss only.	Berry colors, rose, and pinks.	Lip stain or a gloss will play up your youthful soft lips. A dab of a light color or a double coat of gloss will fill out thin lips.
Blusher	Do not use if you will be in the sun. Call attention to your hair and eyes. Keep hair clean and shining.	Skim blusher on lower part of face.	Rose, coral, or peach blusher in powder form.
Special Notes	When you wear warm, sunny colors, ginger, amber, and golden-hued lips and cheeks accent your look. Brown and amber shadows will call attention to blue or green eyes. Your delicate coloring requires early attention to skin care. Avoid sunburn.	Your wholesome looks might make you look younger than you are. A basic wardrobe of bone, yellow-gold, rust, and green highlighted by ginger and honey, with nut-colored makeup accents, will give you the authority you want. Avoid pinks and lavenders for school/office wear.	Your color should be as intense as possible—but still in the pastel range. Play up your eyes and fresh, sparkling hair.
Jewelry	Sporty, casual watches or sports jewelry.	Your favorite pieces can be worn every day, if you wish.	Delicate floral and gold jewelry.

PRIME BLONDE

Shirley Jones, Catherine Deneuve, Lyn Revson, Angie Dickinson, Princess Grace

	Morning/Sports	School/Work/Home	Evening/Parties
Skin Cover	As early as 25 you'll notice small lines around your eyes. Moisturize at all times.	Moisturizer. Even-toning undercoat.	Lighter shade of foundation and moisturizer can be dotted under eyes to conceal circles.
Skin Color	Liquid foundation.	Oil-based liquid. To avoid a heavy look, smooth with wet sponge after applying.	Wear dewy, light-textured liquid to avoid a "made-up" look.
Powder	Light translucent.	Light sprinkling.	Even a slight tan means a change of skin color. Try a darker shade of powder.
Brows	Shape brows from under the brow.	Mix two or three colors together. Eyebrow color can be brushed on.	Keep brows free of powder or other makeup.
Eye Shadow	Brown, beige, tawny rose, sand.	Deep colors on upper lids.	Blend smoky colors around your eyes.
Eyeliner	Smudged color.	Brighten whites of eyes by lining inside lower lid in violet or blue.	Greys, charcoal brown, greens, and teals.
Mascara	Browns and greys.	Two or more colors for an attractive thick, natural look.	Brown or grey for one color coat; follow with black.
Glasses Frames	Change often. Out-of-date frames age the wearer.	Never wear jeweled frames during the day.	Gold, brown, and bright white or metallic frames.
Lip Color	Terra-cotta, mellon, and sun colors in clear shades.	Muted colors, browns and russets, bronzes and golds.	Play up a white or creamy skin with deep and intense color. Lipstick in a tube lasts longest and resists "eat-off."
Lip Cover	Glosses, polishes, gels and sheer shiny color are all young looking, forestall chapping.	Gloss covers can be effective if your teeth are very white. Avoid glosses if teeth are yellowish.	Gloss, transparent or stained.
Blusher	Suck cheeks in, and apply a sunny pink color in hollow. Apply a brighter color on top of cheekbone.	Honey, tans, tawny beiges; warm, pinky browns.	Avoid evening washout look; intensify colors.
Special Notes	There should be one focal point of color for any face. If your eye color is bright and deep, keep the lips light. If lip color is bright, eyes should be subdued.	Don't match nail and lip color, but keep them in the same tone. A tan will give you the opportunity to wear strong, deep color shades; in winter stick to a pale palette.	Avoid an oversexy look. Keep details simple.
Jewelry	Wood, leather, wicker, and natural color gem stones are wonderful and exciting casual jewelry.	Collect important pieces that are exciting and eye-catching.	Pick up golden glow of hair with jewelry.

SENIOR BLONDE

Phyllis Diller, Carol Channing, Zsa Zsa Gabor

	Morning/Sports	School/Work/Home	Evening/Parties
Skin Cover	Heavy moisturizer; pat an extra coat around eye area and neck.	Heavy moisturizer, on neck and ears too.	Heavy moisturizer, lightly patted in.
Skin Color	Creme foundation in rose or beige.	Creme foundation, very lightly applied, only to even texture and color.	Creme foundation in beige or rose colors. Cover neck lightly.
Powder	Light cover, translucent.	No.	No. Powder has a tendency to cake in wrinkles.
Brows	Fill in or even out sparse areas.	Trim long or unruly brows with a small nail scissors. Lighten brows so that white hairs are less evident.	Fill in uneven lines.
Eye Shadow	Beige, nut colors.	Coverstick under eye area to disguise bags. Use eyeshadow only if it is applied with care so that the skin is not stretched in any way.	Beige and nut. Strive for a matte finish in makeup.
Eyeliner	No.	Brown, spice, charcoal.	Grey, brown.
Mascara	Light brown, grey.	Brown, grey.	Brown.
Glasses Frames	Get new frames every two years; nothing is more aging than out-of-date frames.	Surprisingly bright colored frames often are attractive against very fair coloring.	Gold, silver, or frameless glasses.
Lip Color	Pencil or fine lip brush. Corals, peaches, pinks, or rose colors.	Pencil outline; fill in with lighter or less intense color.	Accent on lips with bright warm colors. Pink, red, rose.
Lip Cover	Gloss holds natural lip moisture.	Lip gloss can be applied with sponge tip if evened with a lip brush.	Lip gloss protects and sets color.
Blusher	Rose on plump part of cheeks; rose, pinks, violets, apricot-peach hues.	Avoid bluish colors. Use rose, peach, coral, honey.	Pink, rose, red. Mix sculpture colors to achieve a light-bright effect.
Special Notes	Moisture is needed several times a day. The cells may not be able to hold moisture for long periods.	Heavy or dark facial hair may bother older women. Hair can be waxed away, or facial depilatories can be used.	Don't hesitate to brush face lightly or use a facial scrub. Dead skin is a problem with older people.
Jewelry	This is the only time that whimsical jewelry—like a "Mickey Mouse" watch—might be permissible.	Pearls or any "reflective" jewelry. Antique jewelry, diamonds, and small heirloom pieces.	Antique jewelry, diamonds, and small heirloom pieces. Flowers are great at any age.

TEEN BROWNETTE
Tatum O'Neal, Brooke Shields, Carrie Fisher

	Morning/Sports	**School/Work/Home**	**Evening/Parties**
Skin Cover	Moisturizer on eye and neck area.	Moisturizer on eye area.	Eye, neck, and cheeks; avoid nose or oily chin.
Skin Color	Transparent gel for a color wash, only on cheeks.	Pressed compact for dry areas; water-based liquid on oily areas; blend well.	Rose color for a very pale skin. Avoid a drab look by keeping accents bright.
Powder	No.	No.	Translucent.
Brows	Clean straggling hair between brows, brush with gloss.	Keep a brow brush and a tiny brush or moustache comb with you for touch-up grooming.	Smooth, neat, shining brows make eyes sparkle.
Eye Shadow	No.	Mink, fawn, seal, for blue or green eyes. Violet and blue for brown and hazel eyes.	Onyx and stone shades, teals, moss greens; smudged, dusky and smoky colors are softly flattering.
Eyeliner	Light coat on upper lashes only. Dark brown, grey.	Teal for golden-flecked eyes.	Eyeliner in same hue as the shadow.
Mascara	No.	Brown, charcoal.	Brown, grey, and wine.
Glasses Frames	Match your frames to your hair or contrast them against eye color.	Bright jelly-bean colored frames in green, blue, avocado, and brown are exciting and fun. Try new colors that contrast with your hair.	When you buy glasses be sure they fit your ears correctly. Poorly fitting glasses can cause headache.
Lip Color	Stain in brownish berry, plum, caramel, and peach.	Frost lipstick in bright cheerful color. Brownettes can wear almost any shade.	Brick, spice, orange-brown, and even puce brown can be effective in evening light.
Lip Cover	Gloss or translucent stain.	Lip wands that combine gloss and color on a sponge-tipped stick in spice and burgundy colors.	Rose, plum, pink, apricot, in intense hues.
Blusher	Plum and rose. Highlight forehead, chin, and cheek.	Browns and burnt orange.	Check color in subdued light to avoid washout. Wine blusher is effective—but only for night use.
Special Notes	With blue—a good color for most brownettes—wear plum, sienna, and cherry colors. Masks with clay base can help to absorb oil and prevent a blotchy skin.	Closing pores with an astringent toner will provide a good base for makeup.	You should clean out your makeup case at least once a month. Throw away cosmetics that cannot be cleaned and sealed. Carry a lip/cheek color, brow brush, and pressed powder with you at all times.
Jewelry	Leather bags in mahogany and saddle colors look well with shiny brown hair. Leather and shell jewelry.	Try making your own jewelry from nature: a pretty leaf attached to a comb, or a lovely shell used as a pendant are attractive and individual.	Pretty ribbons attached to a comb.

WORKING BROWNETTES

Princess Caroline of Monaco, Marisa Berenson, Toni Tennille, Liza Minnelli,
Lauren Hutton, Jane Fonda

	Morning/Sports	School/Work/Home	Evening/Parties
Skin Cover	Moisturizer on face, neck, and a double coat under eyes.	Moisturizer, entire face.	Moisturizer.
Skin Color	Translucent color gel.	Color reacts with your body chemistry. If your foundation turns orange it is not compatible with the acid-alkaline balance of your skin.	Matte base in a tube gives skin heavy coverage and velvety finish. Cream and peach tints.
Powder	No.	Translucent powder.	No.
Brows	Arch brows over eyes with the peak or highest point just at the outer edge of iris.	Never shave brows. Cold cream on lids before tweezing will soften skin.	A grease pencil or china marking pencil can be used to even brows.
Eye Shadow	Cover lids with shadow mixed with moisturizer.	Moss, malachite, and soft greens. Browns, toast, walnut, and grey-brown oak.	Chartreuse, chrome, and jade colors play up hazel and blue eyes.
Eyeliner	Upper lid only. Dot and smudge for a natural effect.	Whites, sands, and camels on brow. Chestnut line on crease of lid and brow bone. Match liner to mascara color for thick-lash look.	Raisin, pansy, and violet are effective with blue eyes.
Mascara	Brown.	Musk browns and greys.	Purple, wine, black, grey.
Glasses Frames	Match frames to your hair. Or play up your eyes—green or brown for blue eyes, blue or gold for green or hazel eyes.	Be sure that you check your makeup *with* glasses on, to see how light is reflected in the lenses.	Delicate wire frames or frameless glass lenses; don't wear sports or heavy frames in the evening.
Lip Color	Brick, wine, maroon, copper, russet, sepia, or titian; apply a thin coat.	Apricot and ocher are effective with light coloring. Darker skins take to deep magenta, madder, and puce.	Crayons have staying power and intensity, in burnt rose to deep eggplant.
Lip Cover	Moisturizing lipstick covered with a clear gloss.	Use a combination of glosses.	A lip pencil, pointed with hand sharpener, is easy to fit into a small purse.
Blusher	A translucent gel, several shades darker than your foundation.	Ambers, browns, oranges, pinks, and mulberry should be tested.	Ginger, spice, or warm colors.
Special Notes	Brownette coloring varies greatly. There are several kinds of makeup foundations available. Translucent gels are the most natural but provide the least coverage. Cake base is water soluble and almost opaque.	Brownettes are lucky because they almost always look wholesome—if wearing the correct makeup.	Auburn-brownettes look terrific playing up the reddish hues with lavender, pansy, and violet colors.
Jewelry	Experiment constantly with scarves, jewelry and accessories to see which are best for you.	Gold jewelry reflects warm skin and hair tones.	Gold bracelets and rings look best against smooth, pale arms and fingers. Avoid too-dark nail polish.

PRIME BROWNETTE

Carol Burnett, Fay Dunaway, Shirley MacLaine, Barbara Walters, Sophia Loren

	Morning/Sports	School/Work/Home	Evening/Parties
Skin Cover	Moisturizer.	Moisturizer.	Moisturizer on face and neck, and oil on eyelids.
Skin Color	Liquid in a transparent skin-matched shade.	Souffle or creme foundation. Undercoat in aqua to tone down a too-ruddy skin.	Creme stick in cafe rose and beige. A thin application even-ed out with a sponge should last all evening.
Powder	Bisque powder or a translucent.	Powder in slightly warmer shade than foundation.	Talc is the principal ingredient in powder. A heavy dusting will be drying because it absorbs natural skin oils.
Brows	The most flattering brows balance and frame your eyes.	Avoid thin, overplucked line. Tweezed hairs may never grow again.	Feather brows upward with a brush.
Eye Shadow	Leaf browns, cinder grey	If eyelids are oily, shadow will melt into the crease of the lid; if too dry, shadow will cake.	Egyptian green, Irish green, myrtle, olive, marine, and leaf green.
Eyeliner	Taupe, dove grey, khaki; on upper lids only.	Liner should be applied at roots of upper lashes.	Outline upper lid with browns, bottom with greys.
Mascara	Deep chocolate.	Deep browns. Powder between coats.	Raven, steel grey, wines, and browns.
Glasses Frames	Make sure your frames don't overpower your natural coloring as your hair becomes lighter, select lighter frames.	Gold, brown, and silver grey look businesslike and still feminine.	If your glasses leave a mark on your nose they can damage your skin.
Lip Color	Japanese red, cherry, crimson in stick pencils.	If you like a brush, use No. 3 sable brush from art stores. Avoid licking lips. Corals and warm pinks look inviting.	Frosted in vibrant warm and dramatic colors.
Lip Cover	Gloss in wine and brown over a red color coat.	Gloss.	Gloss. Never touch up lipstick or gloss at a dining table or restaurant; it is no longer acceptable.
Blusher	Rich rosy brown, wines, bronze, copper, mahogany.	Dark foundations mixed with cream blusher can make excellent sculpture.	Warm wood tones.
Special Notes	Perfume oils and bath oils carry the fragrance in an oil base. Woody, green, or spice fragrance is exciting for morning wear.	Eyelash curlers, used only for very special occasions, will not damage the lashes, but should not be used every day. Like false eyelashes, they have a tendency to damage lashes.	Rub translucent white baby powder on your shoulders for a soft velvety look. Use foundation on throat and shoulders to even colors.
Jewelry	A watch and simple ring are usually ample for sportswear.	Scarves and colored stones or beads pick up eye color.	Do not wear matching jewelry. It is dated.

SENIOR BROWNETTE

Betty Ford, Lucille Ball, Marlene Dietrich, Arlene Dahl

	Morning/Sports	School/Work/Home	Evening/Parties
Skin Cover	Moisturizer on arms, hands, and elbows.	Moisturizer on entire face, neck, and ears.	Moisturizer should be applied to water-moist skin.
Skin Color	Liquid or stick. Match the color to your neck as well as your face.	Creme or liquid; a very sheer coat of a foundation with good coverage.	Creme, souffle, or oil-based foundation in a shade that is lighter than the one you wore ten years ago.
Powder	No.	Translucent, lightly brushed.	No.
Brows	Pluck hairs that grow on the temples on outer edges of the eye.	Keep brows a shade lighter than hair.	Keep brows free of powder and foundation.
Eye Shadow	Light cream, sand, beige, with an oil-moisture sealing base.	Stay away from iridescent and vivid green, blue, or violet shadows; they are aging.	White, pearly, and glistening eye shadows are for the bone just beneath the brow.
Eyeliner			Black should never be used on the lower inner rims of the eyes.
Mascara	Powder lashes before coating with brown or grey.	If your face shape is compatible, outline the entire eye in light greys or browns.	Black, grey, coffee, chocolate, wine, blue.
Glasses Frames	Light brown, tortoise, or wood-hue frames.	Heavy frames and a too-close to the head hairdo can draw attention to poor skin texture. Several pairs of glasses should be in your wardrobe if you wear glasses everyday.	Green, light tortoise, and metal frames are attractive for glasses. Don't peer over the upper rim—it is rude and unpleasant-looking.
Lip Color	The sun parches the lips faster than any other skin.	Brown and chestnut, grape, amethyst, for a modern up-to-date palette.	Wrinkles and cracks in lips may come from vitamin deficiency. Rose, sepia, chestnut, as well as heliotrope and plum, can be your best colors.
Lip Cover	Use a sunblock gloss or lip cover. Apply often. Wear lip color to bed, if you like. There are no laws against it.	Gloss.	As you get older the lips become thin. Outline the lip with a darker shade of lipstick, fill in with a lighter shade.
Blusher	Blend creme blusher to temples and ears.	Blusher on the lower jaw and a dark shade under your chin can firm the jawline.	Blusher in warm, mellow colors can liven a sallow face.
Special Notes	Creme perfumes can soften and smooth skin. Night cream, cleanser, and a skin freshener should be part of your daily routine. Soap and water are the best beauty aid all your life.	Don't use red or a reddish rinse on your hair, even if you were a redhead. It only accents your aging skin.	Don't be lazy about perfume. Never leave the house without your own special fragrance.
Jewelry	If your arms are heavy be sure that your jewelry gains importance in proportion.	Jewelry should be carefully selected for balance and shape when it is worn.	Leave the clanking bracelets and charms in your drawer. Don't call attention to your hand if you have any age-spots.

TEEN BRUNETTE
Marie Osmond, Erin Moran

	Morning/Sports	School/Work/Home	Evening/Parties
Skin Cover	Pollution, hormones, and your inherited skin potential all combine to make your complexion. Moisturizer on eyes only.	Too much moisturizer can cause clogged pores and whiteheads.	A skin-tightening mask before moisturizer.
Skin Color	No.	Water-based for oily or combination skin. Ivory, beige or tawny tones.	Use a warm color to overcome sallow, greenish shadings.
Powder	No.	Transparent.	Transparent.
Brows	Heavy dark brows can overpower your eyes.	Brush and train daily.	Smooth to a natural arch; cover with gloss or Vaseline.
Eye Shadow	Light coffee color, beige, creme.	Plum, blues—cobalt, aquamarine, sky blue.	Plum, teal, beige, taupe, brass-copper-bronze.
Eyeliner	No.	Deep blue, army green.	Smoky blue, steel grey.
Mascara	No.	Black, dark brown, navy.	Black, blue.
Glasses Frames	Blue, green, and dark wine frames look wonderful with dark hair.	Don't wear tinted lenses indoors. Match your frames to your hair color.	The new sparkling-glitter disc frames are fun, and right for your strong coloring.
Lip Color	Mulberry, violet, pansy.	Draw lips inside their natural lip line if your lips are too full.	Wine, brown, or even grey pencil can be used to define lip line.
Lip Cover	Transparent or eye creme gloss in a pot.	Gloss can make full lips look fuller, but smoother. Transparent lip-stain in berry and wine colors.	Ginger on lips and copper with frosted highlights.
Blusher	Cognac, rosé. Powder blusher—creme may cause red bumps.	Red roses, coral, wine, ginger; mix and combine.	Muted bronze, and warm autumn tones.
Special Notes	Try a tinted gloss over several colors of lipstick to make your own custom blend.	Denim jeans, in deep indigo blue, look great on brunettes. Excess oils on the nose can look flaky when the oil dries.	Hair grows fastest in spring, and is weakest in the fall. Never brush wet hair. Sleep, relaxation, and a calm nature are the best guards against acne.
Jewelry	Ambers, garnets, and corals are nice as small simple earrings.	Summer flowers and fall foliage can be worn as natural jewelry.	A flower, a leaf, a color of lace all look charming when you glue them to a naked shoulder with surgical adhesive.

WORKING BRUNETTE
Cher, Natalie Wood, Bianca Jagger, Jaclyn Smith, Kate Jackson, Lynda Carter

	Morning/Sports	School/Work/Home	Evening/Parties
Skin Cover	Moisturizer.	Moisture on neck and eyes.	Occasional pimples usually appear just before a big date. Apply astringent or dot with oil-absorbing calamine lotion or clay mask.
Skin Color	Avoid a deep tan, even if you don't peel. It can damage your skin. Use a sunblock cream. Don't try to use pale foundation on a tan skin.	A matte finish gives oily skin a smooth, even, no-shine look.	
Powder	A light dusting on nose and chin will keep your face matte, but natural.	Constarch absorbs oil; it can be used as a powder.	Sparkling white will make you shimmer.
Brows	Daily brushing trains brows.	Your brows should be slightly lighter than your hair. Bushy black brows can make you look old and angry.	Brush brows with gloss; it will make them shine like jeweled frames around your eyes.
Eye Shadow	Blues and greys for brown eyes. Turquoise is especially good.	Shadows must never look patchy; blend with finger.	Allergic reactions to eye make-up can make your eyes red looking and puffy. Eye shadow should be discontinued if this happens. Pablo, the famous makeup artist, likes tiny amounts of green or blue covering entire lid.
Eyeliner	Smudge and dot.	Teal, green or grey on top and bottom lid.	
Mascara	Lightly coated.	Powder between coats, but separate lashes and don't allow them to bleed.	Kohl, grey, chinchilla.
Glasses Frames	Match your frames to your hair. Try offbeat shades like navy, khaki, or wine.	Olive complexions are set off by deep red frames.	Heavy, sporty frames are *not* for evening wear.
Lip Color	Gloss wand, translucent color in earth, plum, eggplant colors.	Transparent frosted ginger, with brown outlines.	With a darker color extend lower lip beyond upper lip at outer edges to produce a smiling lip line.
Lip Cover	Gloss. If upper gum shows too much, strengthen lip by forcing lip over upper teeth several times a day.	Burnished mahogany or nut brown in gloss.	In the summer play up your tan with clear primary lip colors.
Blusher	Lightener and highlighter on bones. Browns and burgundy shades for shapers.	Peach-plum colors of ripe fruits.	Keep your palette in the rose shades or gold like tiger lilies. But don't mix them.
Special Notes	Fresh air and exercise make your skin vital. Walk whenever possible.	Heavy or dark hair on your upper lip or the outer edges of your face can be removed with wax. Do not wash face before waxing, but *do* wash with cool water after. Many Japanese wax their faces daily for a smooth makeup surface.	Exciting, exotic looks are fun. Dry skin does not retain the fragrance of perfume as long as oily skin.
Jewelry		Save exotic jewelry for evening. Avoid any dangling or "noisy" jewelry at work.	Ambers, corals, and garnets in earrings and beads.

PRIME BRUNETTE

Jacqueline Onassis, Rosalynn Carter, Liz Taylor, Valerie Harper, Barbara Parkins, Ali McGraw, Raquel Welch

	Morning/Sports	School/Work/Home	Evening/Parties
Skin Cover	Moisturizer, eye wrinkle stick.	Moisturizer only on eyes and neck. Water-based cake make-up for troubled skin.	A moisture mask before your makeup will keep colors fresh.
Skin Color	Very deep-toned skin looks best with a makeup that provides light coverage.	Excess facial hair can be bleached to blend with your skin tone, or waxed or removed chemically, but you cannot hide it with makeup. A lighter foundation may be best on light-haired or smooth skin.	Broken capillaries near the surface need an opaque foundation or cover-up.
Powder	Translucent.	No.	White or light rose.
Brows	Arch eyebrows gently; brows should be clearly defined, but not sharp.	Most brows need lightening rather than pencil. Too dark brows can make your eyes look small and beady.	Sparkling brows brushed with metallic bronze.
Eye Shadow	Hold lid with fingertip when applying shadow and liner, avoid pulling delicate skin.	Emerald, avocado, deep moss green with gold flecks for brown or hazel eyes.	Yellow, peach, burnt orange, violet, unfrosted shades will open a dark eye and make whites appear more clear.
Eyeliner	Dark brown on top lid.	Match your liner to shadow.	Dark plum, wine, and navy are good for evening eyeliner.
Mascara	Brown.	Deep green, teal, black.	Black.
Glasses Frames	As skin ages it often discolors, smooth olive skin turns speckled—experiment with frame colors that you've never tried before.	Deep tortoise-brown is good on most brunettes.	Avoid heavy frames in dark colors; they can make a mature face look masculine.
Lip Color	Creamy frosted color in a stick; clear colors—red, orange, tangerine, browns.	Glossy-moist shiny lip colors need to be applied often. Keep a lip pot near you when working—in the office, factory, or kitchen.	Violet, pansy, and pinks are best if intense eye makeup dominates.
Lip Cover	Clear gloss; do not blot.	Spice and berry stains in the new wands are an easy way to apply color and gloss.	Transparent in deep colors.
Blusher	Sunny and warm intense shades. Brown creme, blended well, and sparked with powder.	Umber tones from pale berry to deep plum.	Pink, peach, and rose shades.
Special Notes	Air pollution spreads a fine layer of pore-clogging grime on skin. Check your bath shelf for the essentials: pumice stone, bath brush, and nail brushes.	Vigorous movement and daily exercise encourage the elimination of body waste. Don't just sit at an office desk—participate in sports.	Artificial light drains color. Night life calls for vibrant, intense colors. Smoky tones and muted shades in the clothes you wear should be reflected in smoky makeup.
Jewelry	Elizabeth Taylor's fabulous emeralds are perfect with her brunette coloring. Jade can be just as effective.	Avoid dark, heavy pendants if you are exotic looking.	Don't wear necklaces that call attention to your neck and shoulders unless your skin is firm and perfect.

SENIOR BRUNETTE
Dolores Del Rio, Merle Oberon

	Morning/Sports	School/Work/Home	Evening/Parties
Skin Cover	Moisturizer on face.	Let moisturizer set before applying foundation.	Mist face with water, or spray face every few hours.
Skin Color	Skin coverage in tans and ivories evens out color and hides imperfections.	Dewy finish gives dry skin a glowing and moist look. An oily foundation in a warm tone will give good coverage.	Mature skin looks best with a light textured dewy foundation.
Powder	No.	Too much powder cakes on older skin.	Avoid a powdery look; you can blot powder with a slightly dampened cloth pressed to the face.
Brows	Brush only.	For grey hair, smooth charcoal brows. If you use pencil, be sure it is sharpened and clean.	Play down your brows. Trim long or uneven hairs, especially at outer edges of eye.
Eye Shadow	Pink, apricot, ginger.	Grey, sheer white near nose, sunlight blues, greens, violets.	Pewter, dove grey, misty blues. Don't use frosted eye shadows. It exaggerates any small lines.
Eyeliner	Blue, navy, and brown.	A circle of color can reflect and intensify eye color.	Only a very thin liner should be used. If you are not expert, do not use liner.
Mascara	Charcoal, navy.	Black, wine, khaki.	Black, wine.
Glasses Frames		Gold, green, and light tortoise shell frames look attractive with grey hair.	If you wear glasses keep hair away from your face.
Lip Color	Outline with pencil in a shade slightly darker than lipstick. Brown is a good outline color for all shades of red.	If the top and bottom lip are different in color, the lipstick will look uneven. Apply foundation to even lip color—or use different color lipsticks.	Pinks and intense shocking pastel colors.
Lip Cover	Exercise lips singing; it stimulates circulation and retards wrinkles on your upper lip.	Mix and match colors and lipsticks. Use gels, glosses, and pencils to get the color and effect you want.	Dark lip stains.
Blusher	A transparent color gel is good for outdoors.	Blend blushers to achieve a natural look.	Apply lightly. As hair greys, skin seems to lighten.
Special Notes	Actresses who have to use exaggerated facial expressions often show early signs of aging skin. Don't soak in bubble baths: they strip the skin of natural oils and can cause vaginal problems.	Wear protective creams and moisture sealers at all times—even indoors.	Never wipe—blot your skin. Avoid cupid lips; they look ridiculous on an older face. Follow natural line. If your hair is long, brush and comb it starting at the *bottom* few inches.
Jewelry	Pearls have a light-reflecting quality. Select pearls with a pinkish cast.	Don't forget the earring can bring vitality to the sides of your face and draw attention away from sagging skin.	Diamonds are forever!

TEEN BLACK

Janet Jackson (of the Jackson Five), Beverly Johnson

	Morning/Sports	**School/Work/Home**	**Evening/Parties**
Skin Cover	Lightweight moisturizer, thin hand cream.	Moisturizer.	Moisturizer, especially on eyes and neck.
Skin Color	Keep color even, avoid sunburn; use darker than skin tone, matte finish makeup for feature-sculpting.	Water-based for oily skin; mix two or more shades using your forehead as a patch. Do not attempt to lighten skin with cover: even color.	Water-based makeup for oily skin.
Powder	No.	Light cover eyeshadow for matte surface. Copper is good for a healthy glow.	Apply sparkling or fluorescent toast-copper lightly as powder to face and neck. Brush off excess; leave sparkle.
Brows	Even stray hair; do not change shape radically.	Shape arch of brow; upward wing flatters many faces. Fill in sparse or uneven areas with a feather stroke from black eye pencil.	Cover brows with lip gloss and brush to high arch.
Eye Shadow	Plum, deep grey, lightly applied.	Plum, teal, umber.	Plum, wine, grey shadow. (You are too young for iridescent greens or blues.)
Eyeliner	No.	Black, skin tone brown, deep green.	Black liner in a thin stroke at upper lash base.
Mascara	Black.	Black, wine, navy·	Black (two coats).
Glasses Frames	Black, brown, tortoise.	White or very light frames are often too startling with a dark complexion.	Thin gold or silver frames, or no-frame glasses.
Lip Color	No.	Cover lips with moisture foundation. Blot. Trace lipline with pencil—brown, wine, grape.	Cover lip with foundation. Use an oily foundation that you do *not* use on other skin. Outline lip line with pencil. Follow natural line.
Lip Cover	Clear gloss only.	Clear or tinted gloss.	Fill in with transparent lip gloss. Deep red, maroon, grape.
Blusher	Powder blusher for slightly oily skin. Experiment with plum, toast, copper. Eye shadow makes excellent blusher, face shaper.	Plum, toast, copper.	Check lip color effect against teeth. Avoid orange shades, they seem to yellow teeth. Copper and earth tones make eyes appear whiter and larger.
Special Notes	Be especially aware of dark hair on sides of cheek. This can be removed with depilatory cream for a lighter, smoother total look.	Avoid clogged pores and small bumps on nose. Use very gentle washing grains, hot water rinse. Wash face often—five times a day if necessary. But cream eye and mouth area. *Never* squeeze a blemish; black skin will scar easily.	Glamorous means fresh, wholesome, and healthy. Avoid passing fads that will permanently damage your skin. Think carefully before piercing ears, nose, etc. The marks will last your lifetime. Remember *black is delicate*; treat it tenderly.
Jewelry	Heavy jewelry can cause darkened spots.	Heavy jewelry will cause skin to darken.	Lightweight, soft jewelry that will not mark your skin. Make your own "jewelry" from metallic fabrics.

WORKING BLACK
Naomi Sims, Leslie Uggams, Carol Simpson, Diana Ross

	Morning/Sports	School/Work/Home	Evening/Parties
Skin Cover	Light moisturizer.	Color-neutralizing moisturizer.	Color-neutralizing moisturizer in liquid.
Skin Color	Translucent color stain to even complexion tone.	Light liquid foundation, water base on oily areas. Mix several shades from toast to umber until the match with your own skin tone is perfect.	Liquid foundation lightly applied. (Evening makeup means more *intense* color, not more makeup. Evening parties don't give you a chance to redo or freshen up.)
Powder	None, or whisk on oily areas. Even slightly too-light powder is masking and ashy.	Use an oil-absorbing powder. Distribute evenly and lightly over entire face.	Beige-brown powdered eye shadow in tiny containers make easy-to-carry powder cases.
Brows	Shape, brush, fill in with black pencil, brush with gloss.	Shape for grace and balance. A long face needs heavier brows.	Shape, gloss. For a special effect, brush with metallic color.
Eye Shadow	Grey-brown, chocolate.	Beige, umber, grey, navy.	Green, avocado, teal, gold, copper, pearl.
Eyeliner	Black, then line at lash base.	Blue-white lines on inner lids. Line upper lids only.	Khaki, avocado, forest green, white inner-lid liner.
Mascara	Black, dark brown.	Black, wine, navy.	Black, navy, deep forest green.
Glasses Frames	Turquoise, black, bright white.	Tortoise shell, brown, gold wire.	Frameless, metallic wire.
Lip Color	Pencil with brown or plum; fill in with color stain.	Pencil shape as sharply as possible, color stain only.	Pencil outline; fill in with lipstick; reds and purples.
Lip Cover	Protective gloss; reapply it often. Beware of chapped, cracked lips.	Light shimmer, no heavy gloss.	Apply gloss. Blot for matte finish.
Blusher	Toast, rust, and copper, applied very subtly.	Toast, brown, copper. Highlight with one color; shadow with a darker shade of same color.	Plum, dark rose, apricot, burgundy. Use a variety of shades and colors to dramatize your best features.
Special Notes	Fishing, sports, picnics, and water activities are popular. The sun shining on your face will reveal every artifice. Remember—less is more; accent your skin color, don't attempt to cover it.	Carefully analyze your skin color. Is it yellowish, gold, greenish, reddish, or grey? Black skin varies greatly—play up *your* unique tone. Keep skin soft and even-toned with creams; use a skin evener on elbows and joints.	Carry a small white blotter with you in your evening purse. To freshen makeup, press to oily areas. It will soak up perspiration, oil, and grime. A room full of smoke can leave a grey residue on your face.
Jewelry	Natural jewelry—ivory, wood, shell—but be sure it does not rub your skin.	Pearls; small real-gold or diamond studs. Antique pieces.	Lightweight jewelry; metallic fabrics rather than chains.

PRIME BLACK

Josephine Premice, Cicely Tyson, Diahann Carroll, Rep. Barbara Jordan

	Morning/Sports	School/Work/Home	Evening/Parties
Skin Cover	Heavier moisture cream on face, and neck, hands.	Moisturizer on the entire face, neck, and hands.	Moisturizer on face and neck and a double coat on eyelids.
Skin Color	Creme or liquid or a hand-combined mixture. Small quantities can be stored in your refrigerator.	Creamy opaque foundations that will even skin coloring.	Heavy smooth opaque base. Black skin must be even-toned and flaw-free to look its best.
Powder	A cake makeup from theatrical supply houses can be used as a finish.	A powder in rust or rosy shades.	Rust or rose, matched with base.
Brows	Avoid too widely spaced brows.	Keep brows well defined and trimmed, but not too thin.	Brush brows with pearl or metallic shadows.
Eye Shadow	Taupe and dark grey shadow give depth and drama to a dark eye.	Beiges, greys, blues, and deep greens.	Violet, pearlized beige, creamy whites, and butterfly greens. (This is the time to enjoy wearing the most exciting colors.)
Eyeliner	Black, deep brown.	If the white of your eye seems to be yellowing, use a blue-violet liner on the inner lid.	Purple, black, or deep grey.
Mascara	Heavy coats of black; remove with mineral oil pad.	Brown, navy, wine, black.	Black-tipped with metallic or light-catching colors.
Glasses Frames	If your hair is grey or silver, match frames to your skin tone.	Frameless glasses look best on a very small face.	If your nostrils are wide, be sure the lenses of the glasses do not end level with your nostrils.
Lip Color	Brown, plum, maroon.	If lip color seems to wash out easily, coat your lips with a moisturizer base. Rust, dusty rose, deep grape.	Chinese red, bronze, spice; fire engine red is attractive only on lighter complexions.
Lip Cover	Gloss protects lips as well as providing a finished look.	Protective, satin sheen gloss.	Pumpkin, terra-cotta, and rust colors; sparkle lips with a dab of gold-metallic eye shadow just touched to your lip gloss.
Blusher	Use wine, rust or warm brown powdered eye shadow, or deep-color cremes for color and contour.	Earth tones, corals, and rich gingers wear well and look best on deeper skin tones. Avoid yellows.	Sparkling deep sheen. Rich colors—warm wines, creamy colored satins, solid colors in wine to beige shades will reflect color on your face.
Special Notes	A variety of makeup shades should be part of your beauty wardrobe. Send to a theatrical supply house for makeup colors that are not available in stores—even in black beauty brands. Strive for a polished look.	If your hair is dry and the ends split easily, massage your scalp before each shampoo. Set hair on large rollers, or try a natural cut. Do not wear a wig in the house; allow your scalp to "breathe."	Be sure your skirts and slacks are fitted to perfection; avoid pastel colors and printed blouses.
Jewelry	You are a grown-up contemporary woman; avoid jewelry that is too exotic or offbeat.	Classic single watch; gold or silver jewelry.	Pearls with a pinkish glow, and pinkish gold-toned jewelry is always in good taste.

SENIOR BLACK

Mollie Moore, Lena Horne, Josephine Baker, Pearl Bailey

	Morning/Sports	School/Work/Home	Evening/Parties
Skin Cover	Cleanse with grains to rid skin of ashy look. Nourish with natural vegetable oils.	Fresh makeup often; use heavy moisturizer in eye area.	Moisture cream and an under-foundation. Wash face and re-apply moisturizer and creamy base often. Use vegetable oils for nourishment around eyes.
Skin Color	Do not attempt to hide aging dark spots. Match a creme foundation to one shade darker than lightest color.	Creme foundation, for colored but translucent coverage.	Match non-drying foundation to your skin color.
Powder	No.	Very light or no powder. Older black skin has a tendency to look greyish.	Too much power will form an ashy coat; use a shade slightly darker than skin tone.
Brows	Brush and gloss.	Pluck (if only one or two) or trim with nail scissors. Keep neat; pluck white or grey hairs in brows.	Neat and well-shaped brows are important in face-framing.
Eye Shadow	Subtle blue or beige. A dark-colored base can be used effectively on the upper lid.	Beige, grey, light to dark rust, and umber.	Purple, plum, grape, violet, light blue, grey.
Eyeliner	Dark brown, navy.	Brown eyes may become milky and whites yellowish. Blue line will seem to clarify color.	Dark brown, upper lid only.
Mascara	Black, brown.	Black, dark brown.	Black, dark brown.
Glasses Frames	If your hair is silver-grey, try very thin black fames for casual wear.	Match frames to your silvering hair.	Delicate gold wire frames, or frameless lenses.
Lip Color	Plum, purple, burgundy. Use a lip pencil to ensure a crisp, clean lip line.	Use a lip pencil or brush to ensure an even lip line. Lip color in pots, lip stains, and moisturizing sticks protect your lips. You need the color interest to take away from aging eyes.	Bright, creamy colors, deep pinks and dusty roses are good. Terra-cotta and earth colors for the dark complexions.
Lip Cover	Lip gloss protects lips and makes the mouth youthful.	Gloss protects lips from drying weather.	Play up good lips, teeth, and firm skin with gloss.
Blusher	Highlight fullness of cheeks with rosier red color than younger women wear.	If your skin tends to be ashy use cream blusher.	Apply creme blusher to cheeks and ears for a healthy glow.
Special Notes	Your complexion may be mottled, but is growing lighter. White or grey hair will change your beauty palette.	Caramel, apricot, and peach shades are good for colors near the face. People will have trouble guessing your age if you keep your skin moist and soft.	Wear clothes in beige, cream, pastels of pink, green, etc.; colors that were too washed out when you were younger are suitable now. When in doubt, sky blue and white are always suitable.
Jewelry	White, lacy, lightweight jewelry, and an elegant watch.	Pearls, a silk scarf, and bright earrings add a glow to your face.	Diamonds are wonderful on a deep mature skin.

MAKEOVER WARDROBE

Befores and Afters of Accessories

Now that you've learned how to perfect your features and create the symmetrical, balanced and lovely face that you've always wanted, and you've practiced some individual makeovers, don't forget the accessories: the little telltale details that will either complete your new image or make you look strangely out of place and old-hat, even at 18.

While many people may be buying dozens of magazines to study the fashions, it doesn't mean they are copying the latest fashion. The women in the magazines are not *you*. You'll notice that they seldom carry a handbag, get caught waiting for a bus, or are carrying a bundle of groceries, and you never see them getting into or out of a small car. They all seem to frolic through the pages of the magazine, without children tugging on their arms. They are accessory proof. But it is the accessories that make the outfit, the look, and so the makeover. The best-looking makeup can be made dowdy, if you are carrying the wrong kind of bag.

Here are some general do's and don'ts for accessories. They are built on the basic makeover plan—Morning/Sports; School/Work /Home; and Evening/Parties—and they apply to any age.

Headwear

Summer Natural straw with a small ribbon or a *real* flower. Veil for a special look, but only if you want to be very glamorous.

Spring and Fall Knitted beret, cloche, or felt halt. No metallic ornaments, but a small feather on a hat is new-looking and fun.

Winter Hoods in matching or contrasting material, man's woolen scarf made into a turban, knitted stocking cap. (No fur hats; they are old and hot, and cause your scalp to perspire.) A tweedy hunter's cap that you can find in a sports shop or boys' shop. A man's white silk scarf can be used in the evening as a hair covering on a snowy or rainy night.

Scarves

Summer Thin silk, gauzy fabric dyed in contrasting colors; a strip of lace; a small lacy cloth, doubled over as a scarf. A man's large cotton handkerchief.

Spring and Fall Cashmere or silk. No printed silks—the texture of the silk alone should provide whatever pattern there is; some exceptions might be floral patterns or small menswear repeat patterns similar to the type that is on men's scarves, but avoid medallions or anything that has writing on it.

Winter Woolly soft scarves that have fringed edges are nice. Wear several at once; they should blend but not match. Avoid printed fabric; look for natural wool or alpaca.

Jewelery

Jewelry should always be real. It

can be real wood, real brass, real ceramic, shell, or even real flowers, but it should be what it represents itself as. Leave the imitations to people who have the "real" thing in their vaults. The same jewelry is suitable for any season of the year.

Shoes

If you have heavy legs or heavy ankles, don't wear anything around your ankles. Black women should avoid open-backed shoes, unless they are careful to keep any calluses pumiced from their heels. They can stain the edges of their heels if they are much lighter than their skin.

Boots are expensive. The best boots are worth it. Look for boots that are lined in leather, but don't ever wear them in the rain. For rain and snow, buy heavyweight shoes a size too long and one size too wide. Combine these with knee-length heavy socks. It is easy to keep the shoes clean and attractive looking, and rubber-soled shoes are easy to find. If the sock look isn't for you, consider a pair of rubber boots, but take them off as soon as you are indoors; wearing rubber boots for several hours isn't good for anyone.

Watches

Wear either the least expensive, or the very best. The fifty-dollar watch looks slightly blah. Timex makes excellent watches and a Timex, combined with an expensive leather band—my band cost more than the watch—looks as good as any middle-range watch. Change your band often. Use grosgrain ribbon in the summer and leather in the winter. Never select anything but real leather or real cloth; no plastic. A watch, like any other mechanical device, should look like what it is. Don't buy a watch that looks like a bracelet. A man's antique watch can be pinned to your jacket or mounted on a ribbon.

Slacks and Jeans

Jeans are the best slack for the money that you can buy. Buy a new pair once a year, whether you need it or not, and spend time making sure that they are fitted correctly. Go to your favorite jeans store, and if you are in doubt about the style, stick to the classic straight legs, or if you are heavy, the slightly wider leg.

Stockings

Natural color stockings are always in good taste. Never wear anything but sandalfoot stockings with sandals. There should be no mark on your clothes to indicate panties or other undergarments. Pantyhose are probably the best invention since the wheel, or at least since the zipper.

No matter how old you are, you can and should wear textured stockings if you have slender legs. They look fabulous with all sportswear and make any outfit look expensive.

Purses, Bags, and Carriers

Here again the key word is "real." A leather bag must be real leather. Buy the best you can and keep it polished with neutral natural shoe polish. Avoid any bag that has large or intricate brass fixtures or metallic details. They scratch easily and look terrible after only a few months.

In the summer use straw, linen, or canvas bags. Less trim is always better. If you cannot find a nice beige, try a medium brown. Stay away from navy blue or black. Cloth bags should be washable, and dark colors never look right after they are scrubbed.

If you carry a tote, shoe carrier, or canvas or leather bookbag, clean it at least once a month. I think an expensive, real leather briefcase can be used as a bag-carrier by most women and ensures your looking smart and elegant—everywhere.

Wallets and purse accessories should be small and neat; avoid cute gadgets.

Gloves and Hand Coverings

If you keep your hands covered, you'll look elegant and your hands will look young for years longer than if you don't get the glove habit.

If you cannot afford leather gloves, use woolen gloves in a solid color. Mittens over gloves make the warmest fingers possible, and they don't look bad if they are in a solid dark color.

Clothing

For the most successful results in wardrobe planning, select clothes that are suitable for your lifestyle and that will go with the colors of your surroundings. Very few people actually consider the background of the place where they will be, but it is most important. If you work in an office, notice the color of the walls. How do the walls reflect on you, your complexion, and your hair coloring? What about outdoors? The interior of your car? Or even the background of your living room or other room where you might be seen.

For special occasions there is nothing wrong with "scouting the area." If you are to appear at a job interview, make a discreet trial trip to the offices of the company. If you are planning to go to a special restaurant, or if you have been invited to a dinner at a friend's house, think about the lighting and the color of the area in which you will be seen. It will vastly affect your makeup.

Many people wrongly think that wearing dark colors is slenderizing. This is not always so. A plump woman who is sitting in a white room and wearing a white dress will look much more slender than if she were wearing black.

What is well dressed? It is dressed for the occasion in a suitable costume that is both attractive and becoming to you, and attractive to anyone who sees you. Take into consideration the following points:

1 The weather, if you'll be inside or out-side, what sort of protection you'll need from the weather.
2 Where you'll be, the lighting, back-ground coloring and decor, and the general temperature. (It is usually a good idea to carry a shawl or sweater with you in the summer or the tropics. The air conditioning in many build-ings is very cold for some people.)
3 What sort of people will be with you, or what kind of activity you will be involved in.
4 How long you are going to be in the outfit; whether you are going to sit, eat, walk, or ride for long periods of time.
5 What sort of clothing you feel most comfortable in. Do you feel best covered up?
6 What your most attractive feature is. Can you dress to call attention to your attributes and camouflage any flaws you might have?
7 What sort of impression you want to make.

The following are some general rules for making you look more slender, or more rounded. The idea in dressing—as in perfecting the features of your face—is to be in proportion. The above-the-waist areas should be graceful and ap-pear in proportion to the below-the-waist part of your body. Your legs, with your shoes on, should appear to be about one-third of your entire height; your head should be about one-sixth of your total height.

To Create a Narrow, Slender Illusion:

1 Straight skirt (but loosely fitted)
2 Flat pleats, or accordion pleats
3 Slashed pockets
4 Slacks with a fly front or some ver-tical detail
5 Stripes or a vertical weave
6 A solid, subdued (not necessarily dark) color
7 No belt, or else perhaps a matching narrow belt
8 A long scarf, or long beads, or a shoulder bag, very low
9 Medium to wide hair arrangement (unless it is unbecoming)
10 Vertical trim, or no trim at all
11 Opaque or sheer tinted stockings that match your outfit
12 Shoes that are the color of the stock-ing, skirt, or slacks
13 Silks, jersey that is diagonally cut, chiffon, crepe, gabardine, flannel, and velvet. Select clothes that do not bunch or gather and wear your clothes slightly too large; it makes you look smaller inside them

To Round a Thin Figure:

1 Very full skirts
2 Box pleats, plaids, nubby fabrics
3 Large patch pockets, side decorations
4 Contrasting trims and belts
5 Trim, small hats that make your head look smaller than your body
6 Yoked blouses, gathers, and puffs; frilly details
7 Ankle-strapped shoes
8 Light color or contrasting stocking
9 Heavy fabrics; bulky and starchy knitted fabrics will make your body look softer and more rounded
10 A soft bulky sweater matched with a smooth fabric skirt, to make your bodice look rounder and your hips look flatter and smoother
11 Wear your clothes snug and a trifle short, even if your legs are thin

You can be well groomed and always look great for very little money if you stick to classics: a blue denim skirt, teamed with a dark silk blouse or a cotton shirt for spring and fall can be an inexpensive "uniform" that will provide something to wear every day. The same skirt with a pure wool Shetland sweater (you can get one at the boy's department of most department stores) and boots will take you through the winter. The very same skirt—slightly bleached to a lighter color blue, and worn with a white T-shirt and a pretty cotton scarf—is summery and clean looking. For a dressier look, wear the skirt with metallic shoes and a silk blouse—open the neckline and fill with another classic, pearls.

The skirt will probably cost about $20, but it will be suitable for wearing 150 to 200 days of the year; and since it is washable, it will really be very inexpensive if you consider the cost per wearing. Levi Strauss, the classic jeans manufacturer, makes about a dozen different blue denim styles.

There are a lot of clothes that can be bought at the five and dime, and there are some things that must be the "best."

Okay to Buy at the 5 & 10

1 Pants, slips
2 Stockings
3 Denim jeans and skirts
4 Sneakers
5 Sandals (just be sure they are cloth or leather)
6 T-shirts, blouses, etc.
7 Timex watches

Things That Must Be the Best

1 Bras
2 Shoes and boots
3 Handbags

The big expense in most wardrobes is the outer wear: the winter coat. If you can, buy a lined raincoat. Don't settle for one that costs less than $100. If you cannot afford the coat, use a blanket that is made into a poncho. A short poncho can be used instead of a jacket until the snow falls, and the longer poncho can cover a layering of sweaters.

For evening wear, use a dark bluc baby blanket that has been trimmed in satin. A slit in the middle will turn it into a poncho.

People who dress the way I've suggested vary from Ali McGraw to the late Babe Paley. Well-cut skirts and pants and soft knitted fabrics will give you an individual and dramatic look!

Becoming the person you want to be can be easy and it can be fun. The idea of "hard work" ending in beauty is not necessarily true. When you find the look that is right for you, it will seem to come naturally, and you'll be able to achieve the feature-perfecting techniques and image-making easily and effectively.

We all want to be attractive and self-assured and we all want people to admire and like us. But first we have to admire and like ourselves. Any image is enhanced by a smile, a kind word, or a warm gesture. So, with your makeover remember that beauty is only the doorway to your true being and that the most perfect image of yourself comes from being the person you want to be.

BIBLIOGRAPHY

There are many, many beauty books on the market. And some are excellent. The following is a list of books with short descriptions. Unfortunately the list is short; it is because of space. All of the hundreds of books I've read on beauty were well-intentioned and there is no question that the writers wanted to help to make every reader as beautiful as possible.

Bandy, Way, *An Illustrated Guide to Using Cosmetics, Designing Your Face*. New York: Random House, 1977, 96 pp. A detailed description of the techniques used by a very famous makeup artist. Simple but effective methods illustrated with direct line drawings. An excellent explanation of the use of light/dark.

Drake, Ruth, and the Editors of *Redbook*, *Redbook's Complete Guide to Beauty*. New York: Grosset & Dunlap, 215 pp. Using a question and answer format, a complete and clear coverage of all beauty problems and some great ideas for personal care.

Coffey, Barbara, *Glamour's Guide to Health and Beauty*, 2nd Edition. New York: Simon and Schuster, 1978, 248 pp. A complete guide based on charts and the years of experience that come from *Glamour*. New techniques for the sophisticated and healthy looks that identify a *Glamour* girl. A basic reference.

Von Fürstenberg, Diane, *Diane Von Fürstenberg's Book of Beauty*. New York: Simon and Schuster, 1977, 256 pp. One woman's complete makeover, and her philosophy of how to be a more attractive, total and happy person. She tells how to combine beauty and business, and the beauty business.

Pablo, of Elizabeth Arden, *Instant Beauty, The Complete Way to Perfect Makeup*. New York: Simon and Schuster, 1978, 224 pp. Directions for a quick and complete makeup. From the 5-minute touchup to the 20-minute complete fabulous-face, Pablo, a famous makeup expert, has worked with the famous—beauties and others—and made everyone look her individual best. Special section of "most asked questions."

Hauser, Gaylord, *Gaylord Hauser's New Treasury of Secrets*, 5th Edition. New York: Farrar, Straus and Giroux, 1974, 424 pp. A complete book of sensible self-care by the grand master of living right to feel right to look right. Some of the great truths that are never out-of-date.

Sassoon, Beverly and Vidal, *A Year of Beauty and Health*. New York: Simon and Schuster, 1975, 288 pp.
A best seller with good reason; crammed full of information and knowledge, this is the work of experts. Written by Camille Duhe, a wonderful beauty writer, it is clear and supportive, and gives you just the right information to keep you going all year. Nothing better for a long-term makeover.

Livingston, Lida, and Constance Schrader, *Wrinkles*: *How To Prevent Them, How To Erase Them*. Englewood Cliffs, N.J.: Prentice-Hall, 1978, 208 pp.
An active and involving program for skin care at all ages. Many interesting new ideas for the use of household implements as beauty tools. (It was through this book I met Lida Livingston, a great and wonderful lady; a friend and mentor.)

Steinert, Jan Hayes, *Your Face After 30, The Total Guide to Skin Care and Make-up for the Realistic Woman*. New York: A & W Publishers, Inc., 1978, 256 pp.
A makeup expert demystifies makeup. A complete listing of makeups that are on the market and other skin care unguents. Lots of good common sense advice, and a real step forward for the grown woman.

Ford, Eileen, *Eileen Ford's Beauty Now and Forever*. New York: Simon and Schuster, 1977, 256 pp.
An expert on beauty tells how those pretty ladies stay that way. A back section of interviews with some of the great models of the past.

Winter, Ruth, *A Consumer's Dictionary of Cosmetic Ingredients*. Complete Information about the Harmful and Desirable Ingredients Found in Men's and Women's Cosmetics. New York: Crown Publishers, Inc., 1975, 256 pp.
An absolute bible for anyone who is really interested in cosmetics. Fun to read, too. It can save lots of money to know that the ingredients in many high and low priced cosmetics are really the same.

Masters, George, *The Masters Way to Beauty*, with Norma Lee Browning, New York: E. P. Dutton, 1977, 256 pp.
Funny, inventive, gossipy and really delightful reading with lots of icono-clastic techniques. George Masters is the most famous makeup artist in Hollywood. A must for the woman who is interested in looking her sexiest at all times.

Arpel, Adrien, with Ronnie Sue Ebenstein, *Adrien Arpel's 3 Week Crash Makeover/Shapeover Beauty Program*. A Daily Program for Women Who Want to Learn the Professional Way to Go from So-So to Stunning in Just 21 Days at Home. New York: Rawson Associates Publishers, Inc., 1978, 256 pp.
"I can make any woman good looking in 3 weeks!" says Ms. Arpel, and I think she can . . . at least they will know what they cannot change, and what they can change, and how to do it. No fillers; straight-on advice.

Good free information can be obtained by writing to the Department of Health, Education and Welfare in Washington, D.C. And many cosmetic manufacturers are very anxious to work with interested users to perfect make-up and develop new ways of using makeup.

PERSONAL NOTES